Waiting for Baby

Waiting for Baby

One Couple's Journey Through Infertility to Adoption

Mary Earle Chase

McGraw-Hill Publishing Company
New York   St. Louis   San Francisco
Hamburg   Mexico   Toronto

1 2 3 4 5 6 7 8 9 DOC DOC 8 9 2 1 0 9

ISBN 0-07-010708-4

LIBRARY OF CONGRESS CATALOGING-IN-PUBLICATION DATA

Chase, Mary Earle
    Waiting for baby : one couple's journey through infertility to adoption / by Mary Earle Chase.
        p.   cm.
    ISBN 0-07-010708-4
    1. Infertility—Popular works.   2. Adoption.   I. Title.
    RC889.C444   1990   89–33581
    616.6'92—dc20   CIP

Book design by Mark Bergeron

*To my family
and
to the young woman
who gave us our son*

Contents

Introduction

*H*olding this book in your hands probably means you are among the millions of people who are waiting for a baby. Perhaps you have waited with nervous anticipation for several months, or perhaps you have endured years of bitter disappointment. You may have no idea why the basic process of human reproduction isn't working for you, or you may already know why nature has failed you and have tried any number of possible cures. You may be hopeful that the next month, the next treatment, or the grace of God will enable you to get pregnant; or you may be losing hope and beginning to look at having a child some other way. Whatever your situation may be, if your dream of creating a family remains unrealized, you are encountering a major life crisis, and you are in pain.

Finding that you can't fulfill your basic human destiny to procreate is a shocking discovery. Unlike a car accident or an acute illness, the shock of infertility builds slowly, but it is no less startling or overwhelming. It can be even more debilitating than an illness because it can drag on for months and for years with no perceptible improvement and no well-defined path to healing. Because it thwarts our most primal instinct as human beings, infertility is more than a physical disability; it is also a disease of the mind, heart, and spirit. It shakes your most basic sense of yourself, opens you to myriad emotions, and challenges your faith. Being unable to produce the child or children you want affects almost every area of your life: Your marriage and relationships with friends and family are tested; finances are strained; and career plans and other life decisions are put on hold. Life begins to center around the nonexistent baby—trying, hoping, praying, trying again and again, and waiting, waiting, waiting.

In your desperate quest to make a baby, you may begin to lose sight of what you are really seeking. Is the goal to recreate yourselves or to create a family? My husband and I came face to face with that question after two years of fruitless efforts to conceive. Some of you may laugh. "Two years! We've been trying for thirteen (or eight or five)!" Because my biological clock was the proverbial minutes from midnight, we didn't have the time to become infertility veterans. We pursued a course of treatment, but we didn't go to what I would call extraordinary lengths. We did, however, pay our dues—suffering personal pain, social slights, medical tortures, and a financial burden. But we didn't let our infertility destroy our lives or detract from our love for each other. Although we fought and cried, were sad and depressed, and felt hopeless and helpless, we didn't allow ourselves to get stuck in any one place too long. We moved relatively quickly through the infertility maze and came to recognize what was truly important to us—to have children in our lives as soon as possible. Nine months after that decision, we were blessed with an adopted son, Alexander.

Our two-and-a-half-year journey through infertility to adoption was not distinguished by its degree of difficulty or its drama. God knows, we are grateful to have been spared some of the horror stories we've all heard about in waiting for babies, both biological and adopted. We consider ourselves extremely fortunate, and yet we know many other couples who have also found the path to their adopted families easier than they expected. What has motivated me to write this book is precisely that I believe that infertility, while painful and demanding, need not be oppressive and destructive. Similarly, the process of adoption, which seems so frightening and intimidating to the uninitiated, is less difficult than usually imagined and, once accomplished, becomes a completely joyous and fulfilling experience.

Obviously, I am keen on adoption, not as a cure for infertility, but as a cure for being without a child. I have let it share the billing with infertility in this book because I feel that opening up to a nonbiological family is one of the prime issues raised by infertility. Many of you who read this book may already be looking at adoption. Some of you will find, as we have, that fertility treatment is far easier emotionally if you adopt a first child and continue to work on bearing number two. Some of you may feel adoption just isn't for you—nor does it need to be. Sixty percent of couples diagnosed as infertile (unable to conceive in a year of trying) will end up bearing a child by some means. Some of you will grow comfortable in a life without children, finding fulfillment as a family of two.

The first part of *Waiting for Baby* is about our personal process of becoming a family. I share our story with you in the hope that it will help you on your journey—that it will make you feel less alone and even let you laugh at yourself a little. I hope that it will help you get through some of the painful emotions you may feel stuck in and that it will inspire you and encourage you on this difficult path. Departing from our story in Part Two, I offer an overview of the infertility experience aimed at helping you move through both the medical maze and the emotional minefield. Then, for those of you considering adoption, I give an overview of the changing world of adoption and some advice on how to adopt a baby successfully. The information and guidance I offer is gleaned partly from my own experience and partly from other sources. It benefits greatly from my having read several of the excellent books available on infertility and adoption and having talked with dozens of other infertile and adoptive couples, as well as fertility and adoption professionals.

In case you read no further, I will tell you now what this book has to say. The bottom line of *Waiting for Baby* is that *you can have a family*. If you are sure that you want a child, you can and will make it happen. This is true whether you are young or old, rich or poor, married or single. Will it be your or your spouse's biological child? Maybe. Will you be happy and satisfied if it isn't? Almost certainly. If you don't conceive and don't want to adopt, you can make yourselves a family of two, extended by friends and relatives and their children or perhaps a foster child for some period of time. Then, of course, there are always beloved pets, who don't need diapering and who can be left home alone. Having a family is not simply having a child. Whether or not you have children in your life, you can create an environment in which you experience love and wholeness, giving and taking, and connectedness to the whole of human life.

You will have the family you want. I have written this book to encourage you to keep that clear vision before you during this period of crisis. If you do, the process of achieving a family may be somewhat less difficult and painful. Failures will not be "proof you'll never have a child"; they will be proof of your commitment. Disappointments will be only what didn't work along the path to finding what will. Of course, you won't feel this way the day you start your period after an insemination or when the doctor tells you once again your sperm count is low. You will still feel completely discouraged and hopeless; you will still curse yourself for getting hopeful once again. But within the context of your commitment to having a family, hope and desperation are the spokes of a wheel turning, moving you to your goal. Living within your vision, you will know that you won't give up until you are a family—of two, three, or more.

May this book help you clarify your vision and help you make it come to life.

Part One

Chapter One

Trying

 *W*hen I was twelve years old and in love with Pat Boone, I had my future all planned out: I would go to college, graduate at age 22, work at a job for three years, and then at age 25 I'd get married (if not to Pat Boone, then to someone like him). I even picked out the wedding date on a half-century calendar—June 25, 1970. I figured it would be a good idea to be married for a couple of years before having a baby, so I'd get pregnant sometime in 1973. We'd have a girl first, then in few years, a little boy. They would be beautiful children and look like me and my handsome husband. We'd all live happily ever after in a big house by the ocean somewhere.

Thirteen years later, in 1970, I was further from my child-hood fantasy than Nixon was from leaving Vietnam. I had graduated from college, traveled in Europe, gotten a master's degree at Harvard, and was living in the Sixties mecca of Berkeley, California. Two "serious" relationships had not

worked out in the past two years, but I was not overly concerned about getting married. In fact, I was horrified when a
psychiatrist I was seeing suggested I might "just think about
settling down and raising a family." I was in the midst of
having my feminist consciousness raised by attending a
weekly women's group and trying to create a sense of myself
apart from being with a man.

I was also fully engaged in trying to change the world
my generation would soon inherit. It wasn't that I didn't want
to get married, but that bourgeois state could wait until we
had brought about "the revolution"—not a violent overthrow,
but a new age of political participation, social justice, and
racial and sexual equality. For a while, politics was the focus
of my life, but after the murders at Kent State and the increasing violence of the Berkeley movement, I became disen-
chanted with radical activism and grew more and more
interested in psychological and spiritual pursuits.

Throughout the early seventies—the Me Decade, as it
came to be known—I did indeed focus on me, sampling all
the fruits of the California counterculture: psychedelic drugs,
mysticism, gurus, communes, self-actualization courses, and,
of course, sexual freedom. During the time I was biologically
supposed to be procreating, I worried primarily about *not*
getting pregnant. I used the Pill and then a diaphragm, but
avoided an IUD because three friends had gotten pregnant
with them. I figured that if it did happen, I'd get an abortion,
but having no stomach for that particular ordeal, I was very,
very careful. I knew that someday I did want to have children,
but until I turned 30, "someday" seemed very far away.

Even as I entered my early thirties and began to think
more of establishing a career and "settling down," motherhood was still not in the picture. A three-year relationship with
the man I thought was my soulmate came to a sad end, and,
though I had no lack of lovers, for several years no lasting
relationships came my way. I felt sure I wanted to get married

and make babies, but most of the men I met found that idea positively frightening. I guess I couldn't blame them. Commitment, whether to a job or marriage or kids, was not really the name of the game in the Me Decade. From age 30 to 35, I moved about ten times, changed careers completely, and kissed dozens of frogs hoping one would turn into my prince.

In 1980, I was 35 years old, and it was clear my life had not turned out at all as I'd planned. Through meditation, study, and work with various gurus and teachers, I had attained spiritual awareness. Through years of my own therapy, training as a therapist, and working with groups and individuals, I had gained self-awareness and an understanding of my own psyche. As a therapist and then as a writer and media producer working on world hunger and other global issues, I had found work that was meaningful and fulfilling. As an attractive woman, I had explored the ecstasies and agonies of being single—the exhilaration of being free to be with anyone and the bitter loneliness when there was no one to really share my life with. Most important, over the years I had made many wonderful friends, men and women who supported me with love and honest feedback. But despite all I had achieved and despite the fact that independent career women were in vogue, on my thirty-fifth birthday I felt like a failure. Where was my big house? my handsome husband? my beautiful children?

As I approached the watershed of "the late thirties," I felt both desolation and panic. How much time was left on my biological clock? Did I want a child bad enough to have a baby by myself? I tried to focus on my career, reminding myself that I could have as many as ten childbearing years left, that dreams could come true, and that someday my prince would come. But meanwhile, I gave much thought to single motherhood. I fantasized about the sperm donation options: a handsome stranger in a bar? a close friend with good genes? an anonymous jar at a sperm bank? I considered the social and financial consequences: working, paying for childcare, being exhausted, having no social life. I found it hard to imagine a man trying to pick me up at the supermarket while I was wheeling a baby around in the shopping basket, and day care centers weren't exactly the kind of place eligible men hung out. And if no one wanted to marry just me, who'd want me and somebody else's kid? I got deep enough into the issue of single motherhood that I began writing a screenplay about a woman around my age, sort of like me, who decides to have a baby on her own. But I found the only happy endings I could come up with had to do with her finding Mr. Right and getting married. (In my story, it was to her handsome gynecologist.) How else could it "turn out"?

By age 38, I was feeling very much alone and desperate. Trying to focus on "creating" the right man in my life, I compiled a list of qualifications for The One. My list was long and complicated—not just your basic "handsome, intelligent, rich, funny, affectionate," but details like "loves to swim and scuba dive," "plays tennis but not too well," and especially "wants to have babies." I was so discouraged about meeting someone that I started reading the personals ads in a local newspaper, looking for one that matched my list, something like: "Handsome, brilliant, financially secure professional with a sense of humor seeks beautiful, bright, funny, spiritually and emotionally evolved woman, 30–40 who wants to get married and have children." I answered a couple of ads that seemed to come close, but the men behind the print were disappointing. How come their idea of handsome bore no relation to mine?

When the ad men didn't pan out, I took the advice of a friend and tried a new strategy: If at first you don't succeed, lower your standards. I slashed a few qualifications from my list. I found myself going out with several younger men— "yunks" (young hunks) my friend called them—men in their twenties who made me feel young, sexy, and wise. Half-consciously, I began to play little games with birth control—

forgetting a few times to use my diaphragm, hoping, I guess, that something would happen to force a decision.

Fortunately, the something that happened was my prince. On a November night in 1983, when I was particularly lonely and depressed, I dragged myself to a party, mostly to wear some new clothes I'd just bought. When Bill Chase walked in the door, I took one look and boldly accosted him. "Here, I'll show you where to put your coat." I kept him talking to me in the bedroom for half an hour, finding him attractive, intriguing, and single! After that, I let him circulate the party but kept my eyes on him, and by the end of the night we were dancing together, feeling the heat of our mutual attraction. He came home with me after the party, and he never left.

As we came to know each other over the next few weeks, I measured Bill against the qualifications on my list for The One. Some of them he didn't meet. He wasn't a financially secure professional; he was a carpenter who was just getting his general contractor's license. He wore jeans instead of Italian suits. He hadn't made a lot of money or traveled the world. He had, however, spent his twenties training and working as a psychotherapist. He knew himself and he knew people. He was intelligent, sensitive, kind, and fun to be with. He was definitely handsome, sexy, physical, and athletic. Most important, he met the number one requirement for The One: "Thinks I'm the greatest."

Here at last was a man not afraid to express love and receive love. And, yes, he wanted to have children. At a big Thanksgiving gathering of friends, I watched with great satisfaction as Bill tenderly held and cooed at a newborn baby and then romped with a couple of 2-year-olds. Bill, too, had been alone for many years, years of brief relationships that didn't work out. Together, we were like two starving people who had discovered a banquet. By Christmas, we both knew that we wanted to spend our entire lives feasting on each other. On Valentine's Day, a month before my thirty-ninth birthday, we set the date of our marriage: June 23, 1984—only fourteen years behind schedule!

We had a picture-book wedding in the wine country and a magical honeymoon in Tahiti. Our suntans had hardly faded when I began talking about making babies. I knew at my age it could take some time to get pregnant, so I was anxious to get on with it. Bill was anxious not to. Although he liked the idea of having a family, he felt it could wait. He wanted time together as a couple and time to build his construction business. He was afraid that having a baby right away would disrupt getting our own life foundation, financial and emotional, in place. Yet despite these doubts, Bill lovingly acquiesced. He knew the strength of my desire and understood my concern about my age, and more than anything he wanted me to be happy. Yes, he would provide the sperm for this project, but he made it clear he hoped he would not score a "direct hit" right away.

In August of 1984, we had our first experience of making love with intent to conceive. At the time, Bill was supervising a construction project a few hours north, and we met at a refurbished Art Deco hotel in Calistoga. The occasion took place in the Carole Lombard Suite (she had stayed there in the old hotel's heyday). We drank fine wine, lit candles, and joked about having a girl, a reincarnation of the actress, or perhaps a little Clark Gable (to me the sexiest man ever to appear in films). But two weeks later our Hollywood reincarnation fantasy folded with the arrival of my period.

The first few times this happened, Bill was mightily relieved. In a way, I was too. Despite my anxiety about the ticking of my biological clock, I was enjoying our time together and our freedom to play, to find the right house to buy, and to make money and spend it on ourselves. And the early months of trying were fun. We watched a videotape of Lennart Nilsson's "Miracle of Life," the amazing documentary about human reproduction with "you are there" footage of conception.

Holding each other after making love, we'd imagine a marathon of little Bill-sperms swimming furiously upstream, each aiming to be the one-in-a-billion to make it to that big egg at the finish line. We'd visualize that exquisite moment when the winner would penetrate the egg, ending the competition and beginning creation. I'd go about my post-ovulatory days picturing cells multiplying, seeing zygote becoming blastocyst becoming embryo inside me. I'd silently speak to the soul that I felt was choosing to join us in our life, welcoming him or her, offering congratulations on having the good taste to choose us as parents. This I did each month for a few months, ever enthusiastic, expecting to be expecting at any time.

At Christmas that year, we went with friends to Sun Valley for two weeks of skiing. I was excited: We had just put an offer on a house, and I was sure I was pregnant. My breasts were swollen and sore, more so than ever before, and I was looking forward to the most special Christmas gift I could ever receive. I was even a little concerned about skiing. Could a fall hurt our little embryo? I didn't tell anyone, even Bill, hoping to spring a great surprise by New Year's. The surprise came early, red and flowing—I would not begin 1985 as a pregnant woman. I began to feel that something was wrong.

When we returned from vacation, I consulted my gynecologist, who was nonchalant: "Don't worry about it," he said. "At your age it can take longer. Call me if you haven't had any results in six months." The six-month mark came around my fortieth birthday, which we celebrated at a wild party with Mexican food, killer Margaritas, and all my good friends. High enough to fly in the face of tradition, I announced my wish for my 40th year right out loud: "This year, I want to get pregnant!"

To make my wish come true, I was no longer willing to rely on chance. It was time to get scientific about it. I bought a book, *How to Get Pregnant*, and learned that, millions of teenage pregnancies notwithstanding, making a baby is not as easy as it seems. First, male and female must have all systems go: She must be producing an egg or eggs at the right time of the month and have open fallopian tubes ready to receive them; he must have lots of healthy sperm, all swimming in the right direction, and be able to deposit them in the woman's vagina. The sperm have to travel a long distance through a hostile environment (the vagina, cervix, and uterus) to get to the right place at the right time. The egg has to make it to the proper place in the fallopian tube and be ripe and ready for penetration. And all this must take place inside a very narrow window of vulnerability—within twenty-four to forty-eight hours of ovulation.

The name of the game, then, is timing. And the tool for ovulation timing is the basal thermometer, the first—no, the second—essential tool for making a baby. It was fascinating to learn what I should have known all my reproductive life: that a woman can pinpoint exactly when she ovulates simply by taking her temperature.

Well, it's not that simple, actually. First of all, you must shove the basal thermometer into your mouth first thing upon awakening in the morning. You cannot roll out of bed to the bathroom, linger over your dreams, or even reach over for a morning snuggle. The slightest movement can raise your temperature and blow it for that day. So, your very first waking thought must be *the thermometer*. This is a difficult thought pattern to acquire. After forgetting it for many mornings, we strung a sign up over the bed that read "Take Your Temperature!"

Soon it became my daily ritual: Wake up, groggily remember there's something I'm supposed to do. Reach carefully for the thermometer, hoping I won't drop it. Wake Bill to have him shake it down, which I forgot to do last night. Lie immobile with the thermometer in my mouth for at least five minutes, sometimes falling back to sleep and finding it under the pillow or on the floor half an hour later. Then try to record the temperature on the chart, squinting to see the slender silver line (sometimes impossible until after a shower or coffee) and fumbling around for a pen to mark it on the day's date. Observe the daily progress of the arc of connected dots, drawing little hearts over the days we make love, carefully studying the tenth-of-a-degree changes at mid-cycle to detect any sign of impending ovulation. And then, when the period arrives, sadly mark the X that ends a cycle and begins a new one.

The charting of my daily temperatures marked the end of random, spontaneous lovemaking. From then on, we had carefully premeditated intercourse timed precisely for maximum fertility opportunity. My life began to revolve around my cycle as portrayed by those jagged lines across the graph. "Only three more days till we can try again!..." "I'm not sure if I ovulated or not; we'd better make love again this morning...." "My period is due Thursday; God, I hope it doesn't come...." "Oh, damn, it came!..." "Only fourteen more days till we can try again...."

Thus began our years of Trying. "When are you planning to have a baby?" "Well, we're trying." "Are you pregnant yet?" "No, we're still trying." I remembered a seminar I'd taken once in which the group leader gave an example of "trying." "Try to pick up this pencil," he told someone who complained she'd been trying to change something in her life. The woman picked it up and the leader put it back on the table and said, "No, *try* to pick it up!" We all laughed at ourselves, realizing that trying is not doing, trying is trying. As for trying to get pregnant, it is very trying indeed.

After nine months of Trying and months of planned and charted sex, I still wasn't pregnant, and I began to confront the possibility that I was *infertile*. The word itself has always made me cringe. It's not much better than "barren," a term that is blessedly obsolete, or, worse still, "sterile." While the word "fertile" conjures up bountiful images of lush gardens, ripening waves of grain, and trees dripping fruit, "infertile" makes you think of a wasteland of parched fields and bare trees. And "sterile" evokes pictures of clean, white empti-ness—a good environment for surgery but not for the creation of life. From the beginning of time, when God told Adam and Eve to "be fruitful and multipy," childless women were as popular as barren land. Often abandoned by their husbands and sometimes legally murdered, they were accursed outcasts who lived in shame.

Certainly, times have changed, but we have not yet evolved completely beyond the stigma of barrenness. Married women without children are still suspect, and most people will assume that if a couple can't have children, it is the woman who is infertile. So much did I hate that term that I decided to think of myself as "prefertile," remembering the days in the seventies when nonorgasmic women became preorgasmic women—a term that leaves a little more room for change.

As the possibility of fertility problems crept up on me, I began to hear more about—or perhaps just pay attention to —the growing phenomenon of infertility. Some experts said it affected one in eight couples; others said as many as one in five. Clearly it was on the increase, but why? Was it the effect of pollution or drugs such as marijuana? Was it a by-product of the sexual revolution—widespread venereal dis-ease and infections from birth control devices? As I began to read about it, I found that factors such as drug use and pollution have been shown to affect male fertility. I was alarmed by the fact that the average sperm count has de-creased by half over the past thirty years. At the same time, the by-products of the sexual revolution—abortions, infec-tions, and sexually transmitted diseases—have contributed to rising female infertility. But most experts agree that the infertility epidemic is not due to such environmental factors but is primarily the result of delayed childbearing. It is ramp-ant among us female baby-boomers who reached our peak fertility in the sixties and seventies but had the Pill and "bet-ter" things to do than raise children. When a woman puts off childbearing until her thirties she becomes less fertile because her eggs grow older (and thus harder to fertilize), and she is more likely to develop endometriosis (a scarring of the reproductive organs). Also, she has had a longer period of time in which to develop infections related to sex and birth control.

These consequences were not on our minds as we sought to liberate ourselves from our traditional role as wife and mother. The women's movement had freed us to pursue careers, live with men out of wedlock, marry serially, and look forward to a life of having it all—career, marriage, and family. But competing in a man's world for jobs and navigating the treacherous territory of "relationships" was almost more than we could handle. For many of us, the "family" aspect of having it all got back-burner status. Now, as we reached our late thirties, it was coming to a boil, and we were like the crying woman on that T-shirt captioned "I can't believe I forgot to have a baby!"

Few of us knew then, or even know now, about the precipitous decline in fertility that comes with age. A normal, healthy young woman under 25 has only a 20 percent chance of conceiving in any one month. In her late twenties and early thirties, that chance drops to 10 to 15 percent, and by her late thirties, it is down to about 8 percent per month. This means that the average time for conception after age 35 is twelve months.

The averages mean little to the individuals involved, however. As the months passed, Bill and I didn't know if we were just playing out the age statistics or if something was wrong. I was anxious to find out. I went to talk to my gynecologist of several years, Dr. A. I had always felt comfortable with him. He was handsome, kind, and gentle—the type who always warmed the speculum before an exam. I didn't know him well, but I knew he was single and drove a big black Porsche with the license plate PARUNEA, which is medicalese for "intercourse." I figured there must be another side to his sweet doctor persona.

It was about nine months since we'd started Trying, and

Dr. A understood my concern. But since I had had no major infections and had shown no symptoms of endometriosis, he felt sure it was just a matter of time. Our discussion yielded the traditional first prescription for anxious prefertiles: "Try not to worry. Just relax and don't think about it. . . . ."

Try, at age 40, not to worry about beating the biological clock. Just don't think about it while you carefully take your temperature each day and anxiously await each window of vulnerability. In fact, the best possible thing you can do is not care! Give up! This I sincerely tried to do, but giving up in order to get is one of those metaphysical mysteries that I neither understand nor have any idea how to comply with. Okay, I give up. Am I pregnant yet?

When I complained to Dr. A that I was too uptight about my age and possible infertility to "relax," he began a program of procedures to find out if anything was wrong. The first step of the infertility "work-up" is a sperm count, since "the male factor" accounts for about 40 percent of infertility. A specimen of semen is obtained through masturbation into a clean jar and must be taken to a laboratory within a couple of hours. The semen is examined under a microscope, and the lab technician actually counts the number of sperm in a tiny volume of fluid. That number translates into sperm count per cubic centimeter (cc). A high count is around 100 million per cc; a low count, around 30 million per cc. In addition to the number of sperm, the technician looks for motility—what percentage of the sperm are actually moving (they all swim in a straight line to somewhere). Only if the sperm move straight ahead at good speed are they capable of fertilization. Dr. A advised Bill to abstain from ejaculating for a few days before the test to insure a normal count.

The morning of the test Bill produced a "sample," and I carefully carried a glass jar of the precious fluid to the lab. That night Bill told me he had been thinking about how he would feel if he had a low sperm count. In fact, he said he half-expected it, as there seemed to have been so many times when he "should have gotten someone pregnant." But to his knowledge, he had no progeny, born or aborted, a fact that did not bode well for the sperm test, it seemed. I could see that he was somewhat nervous about it. Despite his rational understanding, for him, as for most men, fertility, potency, virility, and sexuality were all linked together, and one weak link could threaten the structure of the male ego.

He didn't have to worry for long, however. The next day the report from the lab showed that Bill had a smashingly good number of sperm with good motility, all headed in the right direction. Bill was relieved to know the problem was not his. Since he didn't have the same drive to get us pregnant right away, he was just as glad that it was "my problem" to deal with. Now the investigative process would focus on me.

About the same time we did the sperm analysis, I had a strange occurrence of my period just at the time I should have been ovulating. The blood was dark and lasted only a couple of days, and I was a little frightened. Dr. A couldn't really explain what had happened but suggested I have a blood test to see if by chance I had been pregnant and miscarried right away. I had mixed emotions about the situation. Should I be happy that I could actually get pregnant or upset that I had immediately miscarried? The test showed no sign of pregnancy hormone, however, but Dr. A did decide to put me on a fertility drug called clomiphene, or Clomid, a form of estrogen that stimulates ovulation.

My cycle charts indicated that I was indeed ovulating but that the time between ovulation and menstruation (called the luteal phase) was slightly short—twelve days rather than the full fourteen. Dr. A said this might be considered a luteal phase defect, which the Clomid would correct. I immediately worried about having triplets, but he assured me multiple births were not a side effect, although there was an increased chance of twins. I kind of liked that idea—abstractly, that is:

We wanted two children, and getting it all over at once might not be a bad idea. (I have since changed my mind about this.)

I religiously took my Clomid, one pill a day for five days—days 5 through 9 of my cycle. Even though it was fairly expensive (then $6 a pill, now higher), I was thrilled to finally be taking some action. Surely we had found the problem and solved it. Surely I would be pregnant within a month or two. An immediate side effect of the drug for me was water retention. I gained about three pounds that really showed on my small body. Two women in my exercise class asked me if I was pregnant.

While I was taking the Clomid, my hopes ran high, and I began immersing myself in information about babies and birth. A friend told me about a fascinating book called *The Secret Life of the Unborn Child* by Dr. Thomas Verny. It presented evidence that at six months, or perhaps earlier, a baby in the womb is a being who feels, experiences, remembers, and responds to his or her environment. What the fetus feels and perceives shapes his or her attitudes and personality. According to Dr. Verny, a psychiatrist, the unborn child is also capable of learning *in utero*. He cited some interesting cases including a young man who found he was able to play certain complicated pieces of music sight unseen. He discovered that his mother, a cellist, had played those scores while she was pregnant with him. Other people, Dr. Verny found, had what seemed to be prebirth memories and could recall the experience of their birth. All this seemed to indicate that there was a great deal parents could do before birth to ensure the well-being of their child. I daydreamed about getting out my flute and starting to play again while pregnant and about listening to Vivaldi with a future musician stirring in my womb.

I was also drawn to learning about new methods of birthing. A woman making a film on "water birth" asked me for some assistance, and I became intrigued with the process. Practiced in France and in the Soviet Union, giving birth in a tub of water supposedly makes for a more comfortable mother and a more relaxed, happy baby. Entering the water environment rather than air is not such a shock to the newborn. He or she stays under for only a few minutes, still "breathing" through the umbilical cord, and is then slowly brought to the surface for a more soothing entry into life on land. I loved the thought of bringing my baby in through a gentle birth in the water. I wondered if such a birth would be possible at my age and whether I could get a doctor to do it.

Each time we made love at the right time, I felt so sure "this has to be it," and I would figure out exactly when the baby would be born—what sign he or she would be. (Oh no, God, not a Leo!) But after a few months of Clomid, there was still no unborn child to enlighten through the womb and no reason to search out a water birth. I continued to ride the rollercoaster of hope and despair. One night, after making love blessedly unprogrammed, Bill and I began talking about what might be in the way for us. So far, we had both checked out fine on the medical front—was there something going on with us psychologically? Although we didn't buy the "not-to-worry" approach, we knew from our backgrounds in psychotherapy that the mind does indeed affect the body. At some level did we not want to have a baby?

Bill admitted outright that although he was sad for me, he was glad that it hadn't happened yet, that we'd had this year to ourselves. The summer particularly had been highly stressful for him. His construction company was growing rapidly, and he was doing jobs that were difficult and challenging—in fact, downright scary. He was working ten to twelve hours a day and couldn't imagine adding a child to that kind of schedule. But it wasn't just that. He also felt that he didn't *need* to have a child in the same way I did, that he could be happy without having children.

His admission shook me. He had been so loving and supportive and I had been so single-minded about getting pregnant, that it never occurred to me he might not be totally behind the effort. He reassured me he was definitely not backing out on the process but suggested that I look at why I felt I had to have a child to be fulfilled.

I was stunned and even a little angry. How could I answer that question? To me, it was like asking how you know you need to breathe. Why did I even have to think about this? Billions of babies have been born without anyone knowing why they were wanted, and millions probably weren't wanted. Why did I have to justify myself? But as I lay awake that night, I began to think about what was motivating me. I had always assumed I'd be a mother. Even in my most liberated-woman phase, I never doubted that children would be a part of my life, that I'd have a liberated husband who'd share in housekeeping and childcare. But the assumption of motherhood wasn't really an answer; I had to go deeper.

What came up first was the feeling of having an enormous amount of love to give. As deeply and intensely as I loved Bill and I knew I would always love him, I still felt I had more to give, more I wanted to give. I felt like an inexhaustible well of love waiting to be tapped further, deeper. And somehow I felt I owed this love to the world. I am certainly among the most fortunate human beings on the planet—healthy, happy, and with a standard of living 99.9 percent of humanity would envy. If I could bring into the world a child who would be loving and giving, creative and productive, I would have, in some small way, given back to life what was given to me.

Yes, this sounded very good—good, clean reasons to have a child, very unselfish and magnanimous. But love can be given to anyone, anywhere. In fact, there are millions of children already born needing love. Why not one or two of them? Did I really want a child to love or *my* child to love?

I had to admit to myself that if I had my druthers, I wanted my own. I liked the idea of a little combination of Mary and Bill—our good looks, good humor, intelligence, and sensitivity. What a joy to see a child running and climbing with Bill's athletic grace, learning to swim with my feisty energy, cuddling a doll with our gentle affection. Yes, I wanted a little us, a magical union of our beings, a tangible presence of our love. We had so much to teach, to share. We knew we'd be good parents —patient, loving, and consistent. We knew, having lived through a time of no limits, the importance of setting limits and of encouraging freedom in a context of responsibility.

As I continued to ponder why I wanted to bear a child, I began to think about my own experience of family. Until I was 7 years old, my family felt like a little bit of heaven. My mother and father and grandparents adored me, my older sister and brother tolerated me, and I felt safe, secure, and loved. Then my father died suddenly of a heart attack, and our fractured family was never the same. My mother worked nights and weekends to keep the family business going, so there was not much time for family togetherness. I grew up very able and independent but also very lonely. I realized that all my life I had longed to have a family to recreate the sense of wholeness I had lost.

I also began to see that the desire for my own child lived at another level as well. I have an ego like everyone else, and like most everyone, I'd like to be immortal. I wanted some part of me to survive, to continue, to play out the human drama however it evolves. Wasn't having a child a way to cheat death just a little, to feel our connection with the future as we do with the past?

One friend challenged that notion, saying that the reason he didn't want to have children was precisely because there would be no future. Could I imagine this planet continuing long in the direction it's going without a nuclear war? How could I want to bring children into a world so obviously heading toward oblivion? His question gave me pause. Having researched and written a book on the nuclear threat a few years earlier, I could not discount his argument. Although the Reagan Administration's macho rhetoric about waging and winning a "limited" nuclear war had died down, the movie "Testament" had etched into my consciousness the unbelievable horror of a mother watching her children die slow, painful deaths from radiation. Even so, I knew I had to learn to live with the nuclear guillotine hanging over us; I wasn't going to let it stop me from living my life. Worse than nuclear destruction would be looking back at a life of choices made from fear and dread.

But underneath all the reasons and justifications for wanting to procreate was simply the good feeling I had when I was around children. I liked these creatures! I liked their openness and joy with just being alive; I liked joining their world of imagination and play. In relation to a child, I felt myself connected to both the larger human drama and the whole of life. Why did I want kids? I liked them and I liked being a family. Wasn't that good enough?

My various levels of soul searching had produced plenty of psychologically sound reasons why I should be pregnant, but we were still waiting for baby. Maybe it wasn't psychology, I began to think, maybe it was just a matter of timing. Perhaps God or my Higher Self or whoever watches over these matters was just waiting for the right moment. After all, we hadn't been married long. Bill did need to focus on the business. Our house was too small now; better to have the addition built first. Money was tight, even with me working; we should become more established. Probably, when we got it all together, then I'd get pregnant. . . .

Meanwhile, to cover all my bases, I forged ahead in the brave new world of fertility treatment. The next step in the fertility work-up process was a sperm–mucus compatibility test. Mucus is definitely not something you associate with getting pregnant—unless, of course, you are prefertile. Then you know that mucus—cervical mucus, that is—means everything. A few days before ovulation, the cervix dramatically increases its production of clear, watery mucus. It serves as a safe, fluid vehicle in which the sperm can travel out of the hostile environment of the vagina and into the uterus. Without adequate mucus, a sperm invasion will never make it beyond the front lines. At the time of ovulation, the mucus should be clear, elastic, and free-flowing. Once ovulation has occurred, it becomes cloudy and sticky. All of this should be easily apparent to a doctor or even to the very observant laywoman, and mucus examination enjoys some status as a method of birth control.

I myself had not paid much attention to the stuff, noticing only the monthly wetness and clear discharge. But I soon found myself trying to grasp some of the goo, stretch it between my fingers (preovulatory mucus is not supposed to break) and generally getting fascinated with its changes. After a week of sperm–mucus compatibility tests, however, I was sick of it.

The test is a postcoital exam, meaning you must see the doctor within a few hours of intercourse. For us, this meant making love at 6:30 in the morning before Bill went off to work. My chart indicated a particular Tuesday would be the likely day, and we dutifully made love. But the cervical examination showed not much mucus and no evidence of sperm, and Dr. A thought we might be a bit early. He suggested we do it again the next morning. Again, an early morning of unenthusiastic intercourse and another disappointment—the quality of the mucus was still not quite right. Come back on Friday, please.

The third try produced some results. The doctor reported he could see some sperm swimming around and invited me to take a look. It took a while to adjust to the various little blips in the slime and finally to recognize one of them as an actual sperm—a microscopic Bill! There it was, head and tail, looking for all the world like the tadpoles I used to catch in the creek when I was a kid. Then there was another, and another. The doctor was amused at my excitement, but for me looking into that microscope was practically a religious experience. Seeing those little buggers made the hassle of the entire week worthwhile.

The next step of the work-up was for me to have a test for serum progesterone. Conducted shortly after ovulation, it measures the level of the progesterone hormone in your blood and gives a good indication of whether you have ovulated or not. The results were positive—a very high level indicating a "good ovulation." But were my eggs making it through the fallopian tubes?

The first procedure for checking to see if the fallopian tubes are open is an uncomfortable and unpronounceable test called a hysterosalpingogram, or HSG for short. Dr. A described the process to me and made an appointment for the following Friday at a hospital in San Francisco. Having checked it out with my prefertile friends, I was expecting it to be somewhat painful and was glad to be in the hands of my gentle gynecologist.

On Friday afternoon, I found my way to the radiology department, undressed and put on that lovely green gown they give you, and was then laid out on a table surrounded with X-ray equipment. I lay there for about twenty minutes as lab technicians came in and out, seemingly ignoring me. I was getting more nervous and afraid. Finally, a nurse explained to me that my doctor had not shown up and that they were trying to page him through his service. I continued to lie and wait and grow anxious. Finally, with no response from Dr. A, I was told I could come back another time or have one of the staff radiologists perform the procedure. I had come this far, so I chose to stick it out.

The radiologist took a large vial of blue dye and proceeded to try to inject it into my uterus though the cervix. It hurt. After a while, it was clear he was having problems. He called in an associate, and they both tried it as I tried not to writhe in pain. The older associate suggested using a smaller needle, and finally the pain of their pushing and poking became terrible cramps throughout my abdomen. At the same time, on the television monitor above the table, I watched the dye flow quickly through my tubes and uterus. There was my reproductive system outlined on the screen, looking just like the diagrams in the book. The radiologist confirmed that the tubes looked completely clear, but acknowledged that he'd had a hell of a time getting the dye into my uterus. He said that the problem might be "cervical stenosis," meaning that my cervical opening might be too tightly closed to allow sperm in, and suggested I have my doctor check it out.

I left the hospital excited that we might have found the problem at last, and a simple one at that. Our hopes were up over the weekend, and I called Dr. A first thing Monday morning. He apologized profusely for having written down the appointment for the wrong Friday, but when he heard the diagnosis, he said cervical stenosis seemed unlikely. It is a condition usually characterized by intense pain during menstruation. I usually had some mild cramps, but nothing horrible. Still, he said would check me out during my next period.

When he checked out my cervical opening, he said he couldn't really conclude that stenosis was the reason I wasn't getting pregnant, but it might be a contributing factor. Probably there was some sort of cervical problem as well as the possible "luteal phase defect" for which I was taking Clomid. He also reminded me that the HSG is not a conclusive test for determining tubal problems. It does not show adhesions inside and outside the tubes, so scarring from infections and endometriosis might not be detected. All the HSG could tell us was that my tubes weren't blocked and that "the plumbing looks fine," but it would take an operation called a laparoscopy to provide a reliable diagnosis. He didn't feel this was the time for surgery, but instead he referred us to a fertility specialist. The next most logical treatment, he said, was to try intrauterine insemination, and the doctor he referred us to was considered the top insemination expert in the area. We called immediately and found we couldn't get an appointment until the following February, five months away.

Chapter Two

❦

Trying Anything

A year had passed, and we
had now joined the ranks of couples officially considered "infertile"—those who have tried unsuccessfully to get pregnant
for more than twelve months. I admitted to myself that we
had a problem, but I was sure it was one I could solve
if I put my mind to it. I would overcome it the way I had
any other problem in life: by learning and doing everything I
could. I went to the library and got out books and articles
on infertility. I bought magazines that featured articles on
"Dramatic New Breakthroughs in Infertility." I gave them to
Bill to read, too, but usually they sat on his desk for weeks.
"Just tell me what it says," he'd say, and I'd summarize. He
learned by osmosis, still believing our pregnancy was only a
matter of time. I wasn't so sure and began talking with everyone I knew who was a member of the anxious fraternity of
prefertiles.

I turned first to my friend Nancy,* who was a couple of years older than I and who had been trying to get pregnant for over a year. A big, attractive blonde who had once been a brown belt in karate, Nancy had been married to Bart for five years. He was handsome and young, thirteen years her junior, but the age difference apparently had had no effect on their very happy and stable marriage—until they decided to have a child.

Nancy had had an abortion when she was 20 and had not been pregnant since. After they'd been trying for a year or so, she and Bart began the fertility work-up (a traumatic experience for Bart, who found he "couldn't get it up" for the sperm count test). They had done all the tests we had, plus a laparoscopy, but still had no diagnosis. Spontaneous sex was rare for them, although they actually followed a friend's suggestion to "do it in the back seat of a car."

They were beginning to question themselves. "Is it that we really don't want to have kids?" Nancy asked. "I don't know, maybe we just don't have a really clear intention to be parents." She admitted that she had always felt she could be happy without children, but she didn't want to deny the experience to Bart, who came from a large family. She wondered if she'd gone from being ambivalent about it to wanting it more because it was something she couldn't have. Both of them were feeling the pressure in their marriage, Bart questioning if the infertility was because Nancy didn't really want to have kids and Nancy feeling resentful that all the effort of fertility treatment was falling on her. As their lovemaking became increasingly programmed and they began to focus on intrauterine insemination, Bart got to the point of not even caring about sex. "I'm never looking into Nancy's eyes," he said. "It's always the eyes of the Playmate of the Month."

---

*All of the people referred to by first name only are real people. Their names have been changed, however, for the purpose of confidentiality.

Nancy and I commiserated on the phone when our periods started. Over lunch we complained to each other about how unfair it was—all the women who didn't want kids but seemed to have no problem getting pregnant. And here we were in the prime of our lives—healthy, happy, stable, and with so much to give and share. We had it all, but we were unable to create the beings we wanted to share it all with. Oh well, at least we could have another glass of wine....

Another source of information and gossip was my exercise studio, an upscale scene with a parking lot littered with Mercedes, BMWs, Audis, and Porsches. Some of the aerobicizers there knew the meaning of the saying "You can't be too thin or too rich" and wore their Rolex watches, gold necklaces, diamonds, and pearls right along with their perfectly coordinated leotards, tights, and legwarmers. Three times a week I braved the most macho classes, every day vowing I'd stop eating ice cream and live on vegetables and fruit. In the dressing room before and after class, women who knew I was trying to get pregnant offered advice and told stories of friends who had done this and done that, who had been successful or not.

It was in the Monday-Wednesday-Friday advanced class that I became reacquainted with Beverly, a woman I had known years before when we both lived on the East Coast. She was now a successful psychotherapist, slim and beautiful at age 38, an energetic woman who hardly seemed to sweat during the workouts. When I told her about trying to get pregnant, she told me she was in the same situation only worse—she had miscarried twice.

Before the miscarriages, she said, she had been somewhat ambivalent about having a child, not sure she was really the maternal type. "Family" was somewhere out there—not the dream of her life, just sort of "the next thing to do." But having been pregnant twice and lost two babies in the first trimester, she was devastated, and now she felt completely driven to have a child. Her first two pregnancies had occurred easily, in the first and second month of trying. It had been several months now, and she and her husband were undergoing fertility treatment.

Beverly tried to play down her miscarriages, telling me that first and even second miscarriages in the first trimester are "normal" and that about a third of women over 35 miscarry the first time, but I knew she was in pain and deeply worried. I couldn't help but identify with her anguish and fear. Getting pregnant and losing the baby had not seemed a real possibility until I got to know Beverly. I began to imagine what the chances were for me in my early forties and got good and scared.

I talked frequently on the phone with my best friend, Anna, who lives in North Carolina. Since we met in college, our friendship had remained extraordinarily close, even though we almost always lived a continent or even an ocean apart. She had married an artist from Morocco. They had lived and traveled in Africa, crossing the Sahara in a Land Rover twice, but had settled down in her hometown to raise a family. Her childbearing had gone according to plan: first a beautiful daughter and five years later a handsome son. They were the perfect family, and Anna, who was passionate about everything in life, gave herself fully to being a mother. Even though she was an early feminist, she now had a religious fervor about women staying home to raise their children.

As our phone conversations started focusing on my fertility problems, Anna kept me informed about two of our mutual friends in North Carolina. Elaine, who had gone to college with me, was a brilliant, driven woman who had graduate degrees in theology and nursing and was now the administrator of a nursing home. Like me, she had found her true love late in life. She and Jim started Trying when she was 35, and during the past five years, she had had several operations to clear up endometriosis.

Endometriosis was a word I had barely ever heard until the past few months, and now it sounded almost as ominous to me as the "C-word"—cancer. The "E-word" can be just as devastating in terms of fertility; it is a leading cause of infertility in women, affecting over 15 percent of us. Usually it occurs in women between 30 and 40 who have not borne a child, and it renders half its victims infertile.

In endometriosis, cells from the endometrial lining of the uterus get into the pelvic cavity and begin to grow in the fallopian tubes, the ovaries, or other places they do not belong. Responding to menstruation signals, they are sloughed off but have no place to go. They then become inflamed and leave scar tissue that interferes with the normal functioning of the reproductive organs. Most women who have endometriosis experience severe cramps around their period, but mild cases may produce no recognizable symptoms. Elaine had not had pelvic pain, but a laparoscopy revealed the problem. Treatment with a drug called Danazol (a form of male hormone that stops ovulation) and microsurgery cleared the scar tissue, but a year later it returned. Apparently, there is no cure for endometriosis; it can only be contained.

Each time I learned about a new cause of infertility, I wondered if that was the one affecting me. Could I have endometriosis even if I didn't have severely painful periods? Could I have had pelvic inflammatory disease sometime in my life and not known it? Could I be "allergic" to Bill's sperm, producing antibodies that killed them off? Could I have some bacterial infection like Chlamydia? Dr. A assured me that he saw no sign of infection and that Bill's sperm was alive in my mucus. No, he didn't think I had endometriosis, but I should wait to talk to the fertility specialist. I felt impatient and afraid.

I felt more afraid when Anna called me about another mutual friend, Susannah. She and her husband Ed were both about my age, and I had known them since they were married right after college. A more wonderful pair of human beings you could not imagine. As a college campus minister, Ed had continued his Sixties activism into the eighties, working hands-on on social issues most of us just contribute money to. Susannah was also an inspiring and giving person who worked with underprivileged children and tutored prisoners. They both loved children and had wanted a family for many years, but they were unable to get pregnant. Ed had a low sperm count, and treatment had yielded no results. Finally, they adopted a beautiful little girl but kept on trying for a second child.

I happened to be with Susannah the night she decided to give up on getting pregnant. We were at a seminar together where we saw a film of a natural childbirth—pain, panting, some screaming, and then cries and tears of ecstasy. On the way home, Susannah was very quiet. When she finally talked, she said she had been profoundly moved. Watching the film, something inside of her had shifted, and she knew she was willing at last to let go of giving birth. She felt she had finally accepted her infertility; she would not hope and cry about it anymore. Three months later, Susannah was pregnant. She and Ed and all their friends were ecstatic. There was at least one clear piece of evidence on the side of the old notion, "Give it up and then it will happen."

But there was no happy ending to this miraculous story. Two weeks before the baby girl was due, a freak twisting of the umbilical cord choked off her life. Susannah and Ed buried their baby and tried to live with their grief. Their tragedy shook me to the core. It was not merely the injustice of such a senseless, cruel blow to two beautiful people; it was also the realization of the precariousness of our dreams. Even if they come true, they can still die. And in the fifth decade of life, a woman's dreams of childbearing face a treacherous path toward realization. For the dream to come true, being a good person isn't enough; you have to be lucky.

I did know of a few lucky ones. I knew Sandy, already the mother of two grown children, who had had two miscarriages while trying to get pregnant with her second husband.

Finally, she thought she was beginning menopause but, to her surprise, found that she was pregnant. At age 47, she gave birth to a beautiful son. I also knew Diana, who had developed pelvic inflammatory disease from a Dalkon Shield, the birth control device linked to infection and infertility among tens of thousands of women. Diana went through several surgeries, but her doctors said her reproductive organs had been too badly damaged. They said the chances were "one in a million" that she'd ever bear a child. Three years after adopting a baby boy, she gave birth to a girl. Another friend, Lana, had had her endometriosis corrected by laser surgery and had gotten pregnant just a couple of months later—on Mother's Day.

It was heartening to know of some success stories and also to read that 40 or 50 percent of couples who get the appropriate treatment for their problem are able to have a child. Even among those who do not have any treatment, there is a "spontaneous cure" rate of about 10 percent in the first year and 5 percent in the second year.

I tried to concentrate on the lucky ones as I awaited fertility treatment or a treat from the Universe—full breasts and a late period. I imagined that if I did get pregnant, I would know right away, within a few days. I questioned every woman I knew who had a baby about when and how she knew. A couple of friends told me they were aware of the very moment of conception, that they actually "felt it psychically" after making love. I hated them. I felt better when a couple of women told me they had no idea they were pregnant until their period didn't show up; it gave me hope throughout the entire latter part of my cycle.

My cycle had shifted somewhat from taking the Clomid, and, rather than a regular twenty-eight days, it now lasted anywhere from thirty-two to thirty-five days. My hope and anxiety began to build around day 28 and would gain momentum each time I went to the bathroom and found no sign of my period. By day 32 or 33, I lived in a state of perpetual tension, thinking about it only around a hundred times a day, afraid to go to the bathroom, afraid to say anything to Bill or anyone for fear I would jinx myself. When the blood began to flow, I felt wretched. Each occasion felt like a little funeral, a mourning for the death of someone who had never existed. If I could, I'd have a good cry; otherwise I'd mope around. Bill could tell the minute he got home. "You started," he'd say and hold me close, letting me whine about how unfair it was, how angry I was, how sad I felt. The depression would last a few days and then start fading into hope again as we headed toward the next month's "prime time."

The roller coaster ride began to wear on Bill as well, but he felt a strange mixture of emotions. One feeling was relief, the sense that it was better to wait a while longer for a baby to come into our lives. Another was discouragement because our failure to conceive again and again did seem to indicate a problem. He was also sad because I was so unhappy and upset, but at times he was angry at me for getting so down. He would remind me it was probably a function of our ages, and that "it will happen when it happens." He knew that was easy for him to say, since he felt more like an observer than a participant in the biological drama going on. It felt good to be able to talk to him about it and to know that, even when he was annoyed with me, I could still count on him for love and consolation. I was grateful that I could let him have his own feelings without feeling threatened.

As my life continued to revolve around my cycle, I began to confront the various pains, large and small, of being infertile in a fertile world. Despite growing awareness of the issue in recent years, infertility is still a subject not unlike death or a fatal disease. Everyone feels sorry for the couple involved, but people hesitate to talk about it; few know what to say or how to be sensitive and caring. Truly, it is a very personal issue, which some people choose not to share with others. If you don't talk about it, people may assume you don't want children. If you are open about it, as Bill and I were, you risk some annoying comments and some painful situations.

One of the most common responses is "I'll bet you're having fun trying." Ha ha ha. Truth is, programmed intercourse usually isn't hot sex. Not that it isn't enjoyable, but it's hard to abandon yourself to lovemaking when you're thinking all the time, "Please, please let this be the time." Another common response is "Just relax and it will happen"—as if tension were the root cause of infertility. If that were so, there would surely be far fewer teenage pregnancies.

Often, people are incredibly insensitive, like a man I worked with on a project. The father of three children, he would brag about how potent he was: "I can knock up my wife practically by looking at her." His attitude intimated that Bill was less than a man, and more than once he suggested, half-jokingly, that I should give him a crack at it. I wanted to slug him. Women, too, can be unconsciously hurtful, almost bragging about the number of abortions they've had or about how easy it is for them: "It happens if I just *think* about it." Often, mothers laugh nervously and tell you that you don't really want kids. "They really cramp your style. Are you sure you really want all this hassle?" Sometimes, people want to protect you. My sister-in-law didn't want to call us right away to announce her second pregnancy for fear she'd upset us. One friend thought he was being encouraging, I guess, by asking every time he called, "Are you pregnant yet?"

From the beginning, we were quite open and frank with our families, letting them know we were trying, keeping them posted on the medical developments, and sharing our feelings about the lack of results or even a diagnosis. We were fortunate that all the would-be grandparents, aunts, and uncles were kind and understanding, as family expectations can put enormous pressure on a couple. Some families don't talk about it at all, as if infertility were shameful, a skeleton in the closet.

Nancy told me that Bart's parents never mentioned it to them, even though she knew they were anxious for grandchildren. Other couples said their relatives were constantly asking about it—"So what's wrong with you two?"—and making comments like "I certainly hope to have grandchildren before I die."

During visits to Bill's sister and brother-in-law in Los Angeles, I would often get choked up watching Bill play with our 4-year-old nephew, George. They'd race around the house yelling "Transformers transform!" turning alternately into robots, spaceships, and monsters. Bill would dangle George by his feet, tormenting him with tickles, and would never fail to crack him up with his Donald Duck voice. I loved to watch their horseplay and longed to hear those squeals of delight in my own home. A few months after nephew number two arrived, we were treated to the complete birth on videotape. My emotions swirled as we watched. It sure didn't look like fun, but when Dean's head pushed through and when Barbara held him in her arms, I fought back tears of sadness and envy.

We were luckier than most prefertile couples, however, since our nieces and nephews lived far away, and few of our close friends had children who were not already teenagers or beyond. For couples who have to be around friends and relatives with babies and children, contact can be painful, particularly during holidays. You think you'll cry if another adorable trick-or-treater comes to your door dressed as a ballerina or Superman. Thanksgiving with the family can be an ordeal when you have no one to sit at the kids' table, no one to brag about—how well she eats, how fast he got toilet trained, or all the new words she's saying now.

Christmas, the holiday for children, is the hardest on prefertiles. On shopping trips they are everywhere, running around stores and climbing up on Santa's knee. And so are the toys—mechanical contraptions that turn into everything but the kitchen sink, furry magical creatures from the netherworld, and dolls that look like real babies (should you buy yourself one?). At home, the decor is beautiful, but everything is too clean and tidy. No little stockings to hang over the hearth. No toys to wrap. No one but you to eat all the cookies. No squeals of wonder and delight on Christmas morning. Beverly and her husband David found family gatherings almost impossible to bear and decided one year to go skiing instead.

Bill and I felt the holiday blues most strongly at a festive Christmas open house held annually by some friends at their huge house in San Francisco. We circulated upstairs, drinking, eating, and small-talking with the adults, and then went downstairs, a large area transformed into a Christmas wonderland for kids. Santa's elves were the babysitters for the most beautiful children you could imagine, dozens of them decorating cookies, painting faces, snuggling up to Santa, and munching on miniature hamburgers and hot dogs. The scene was a wild one, and most parents were eager to drop off the kids and get back upstairs to the champagne and adult feast. But Bill and I lingered in Santaland, admiring, envying, longing for the day we could watch our own child crawl up on Santa's knee and whisper in his ear. We stood there somewhat subdued, feeling like outsiders, and then headed back upstairs to the grown-ups. The party wasn't quite the same afterwards.

During prefertility, you have to be wary of such gatherings, of unexpected upsets such as diaper commercials on TV, and especially of grocery stores, a favorite hangout of mothers and babies. Sometimes I felt like avoiding them completely, doing my shopping in the early evening and taking care not to wheel down the "baby aisle." Other times I would ignore my shopping list just to follow a little cutie around the store. Baby craving produces strange approach–avoidance situations: Seeing babies makes you sad, but you want to be around them. You ogle them on the street as you once did hunky guys. You think all children are adorable, no matter how ugly or obnoxious they are. You boldly approach babies anywhere anytime to coo at them and feel a little hand curl around your finger. You

stare longingly into cars with baby seats and sigh with envy
at those "Baby on Board" stickers—the yellow badge of the
fertile. You feel completely envious of pregnant women, you
hate them, and yet you are in awe of them, almost wanting to
be touched by them, blessed and sanctified.

I actually fared pretty well during a baby shower for a
friend, as I was still confident then that I, too, would soon be
the recipient of all those adorable, expensive outfits babies
outgrow so quickly. But I knew if our infertility stretched on,
baby showers were a surefire thing to avoid. I wondered, too,
how I would react if my friend Katherine got pregnant before
I did. She and her husband Vern had just decided to go for
it, and I could already feel the envy building. I just knew she'd
get pregnant right away and I'd hate her. Nancy had told me
that her and Bart's best couple friends had recently had a
baby, and though at first it was fun babysitting and hanging
out with the three of them, it got to be very painful after a
while. Katherine and Vern were our best couple friends—
would a baby come between us?

Because Bill and I were quite open about our fertility
problems, our friends knew what we were going through and
were very supportive. In fact, we were deluged with advice:
"Bill should not come for two weeks; then, after you do it,
stand on your head or hold your legs up for 20 minutes...."
"You should stop doing those aerobic classes. They jiggle
things around too much...." "Eat lots of raw oysters and take
a lot of vitamin E...." "You guys shouldn't take hot tubs, they
lower Bill's sperm count. And he should wear boxer shorts.
You know what they say: 'Keep a cool crotch.'..." "You guys
just need to get away from it all—take a vacation...." "Try
meditating on being receptive—just let it happen...." "I just
heard about this acupuncturist called the 'Baby Wizard.' Three
of his patients got pregnant after years of trying...." "Why
don't we have a fertility ceremony at the full moon? Everybody
bring fertility symbols...."

Feeling stymied in the medical category, I felt ready to try just about anything, from old wives' tales to New Age metaphysics. Despite the doctor's assurance that it would make no difference whatsoever, I propped my legs up after intercourse, avoided hot tubs, and ate up the vitamin E. I switched to low-impact aerobics classes and started swimming instead of running. When a friend called to tell me about a psychic she had seen, a woman from Los Angeles who had given her an accurate and "powerful" reading, I started thinking about investigating infertility at the psychic level. Was there something going on unconsciously that was preventing me from getting pregnant?

I had consulted psychics on several other occasions in my life and had usually found the information from the "readings" useful, if not terribly accurate. I don't know how many times I was told I'd get married in the next year—year after year. Often, however, the messages about my emotional state and the direction in which I needed to grow were very helpful. I'm not quite sure what I believe about people who claim to be psychics, perhaps they do indeed see into the past and future, or perhaps they are just highly intuitive and able to "read" your emotional state. Perhaps it's all mumbo jumbo. I am not a true believer in psychic phenomena, but I am not a complete skeptic, either. There are too many mysteries in life for me to claim to know anything with certainty. I prefer to be open to it all and take what's useful to me. Bill was a bit more skeptical because he had never been to a psychic before. Out of curiosity, he consented to our seeing her together.

We climbed down steep steps through dense summer fog to meet her one evening. She called herself Angela, one name only, and was a quite attractive woman in her forties. In the center of her loose lavender blouse hung a large crystal pendant on a gold chain. She sat in the lotus position on a couch and asked us a few questions in a soft Southern accent. Then she went into some sort of a trance, and I was invited to ask her questions. Right away, I said that we wanted children, that we'd been trying for a year, and was there something in the way of our conceiving that we weren't aware of? There was silence for a few moments before she spoke softly but emphatically. She told me that I had a great deal of fear associated with having children and that this was an opportunity to heal the fear. The fear, she said, came from experiences that had taken place in past lives, lives that I could not remember consciously but that still affected me. There is really no such thing as time, she said, and we could return to those incidents now. In the realm of "no time," we could change them.

I wasn't sure what she was talking about but expressed my willingness to go through the process with her. Bill sat still and expressionless, and I tried to imagine what was going on in his mind. But soon I was swept into the drama that unfolded. Angela took me through three "past lives" in which I had lost children under brutal circumstances. In one life, I was a Japanese peasant forced to flee warring samurai who butchered my son and daughter. In another, I was an American frontier settler, and it was Indians who murdered my three children. In a third life, presumably in the nineteenth century, my only child died of smallpox.

In each of these incidents, Angela "rewrote" or rather renarrated the story for me, asking me to visualize the situations differently. She described them as if we were watching a movie: we managed to escape the samurai; we moved from the settlement before the Indian attack; the child recovered from smallpox. All's well that ends well. She then declared me healed and told me that Bill and I would have at least one child, but she didn't give any time frame for her prediction. Relax and don't worry about it (yes, that again) and "let it happen." She acknowledged that we both did indeed want children and that we would be excellent parents. We then went on to other subjects, about which she was also encouraging.

As we climbed back up the stairs, I felt a bit eerie. The past life experiences didn't seem very real to me; I didn't connect with them emotionally. Still, they were very interesting, and who knows, the "healing" might somehow make a difference. Back home, Bill was less generous. He felt that "past lives" were at best a metaphor for accessing the unconscious. If the stories had not felt real to me or triggered an emotional reaction, it was probably a useless exercise—a waste of our time and a hundred dollars. "Forget trying to figure it out," he said. "You're going to get pregnant. We'll do whatever we have to to make it happen."

What I did next was follow up the leads on the acupuncturist known as the "Baby Wizard." I talked on the phone to two women, both of whom had gotten pregnant after years of trying and credited their success to several months of acupuncture treatments. I had had acupuncture treatments myself several years before for a chronic condition and felt it was helpful. I found the Chinese approach to medicine a highly sensible one. They see the body as a whole system, a delicate balance of energies. Pain or disease indicates an imbalance somewhere in the system. Acupuncturists don't just treat the symptom but aim to create a systemic balance in which the body can heal itself. The five main energy systems flow on paths throughout the body that are called meridians. Acupunturists insert very slender needles at points on the meridians in order to stimulate or calm the energy flow. Surprisingly, the needles are not painful, and I had found the treatments to be very relaxing.

I was enthusiastic when I called Dr. Wu.* Although his English was barely comprehensible, I understood that he felt he could help me as long as my tubes weren't physically blocked. I assured him the HSG test had showed them open and that I was eager to begin treatment right away. A few days

---

*Not his real name.

later, I was scouring the outskirts of Chinatown for a parking place, an hour-long project in itself. Walking down the steep hill in search of Dr. Wu's office, a fairly grungy looking duplex, I felt a surge of hope. Inside, I was less optimistic. The apartment/office was hot and dirty, the bathroom smelled less than fresh, and the three people waiting with me in the front room looked strange. After a while, a long-haired young Caucasian man informed me reverentially that Dr. Wu would see me in a few minutes. I leafed through a two-year-old magazine and a pamphlet about Chinese herbs. About twenty minutes later, the young man led me to an "examining room," a small dark room with two tables only a few feet apart and a window facing a brick wall. The room was divided by a curtain, behind which Dr. Wu (I presumed) was treating a mother and her young child. The child was squirming, the mother was trying to calm him, and I was getting more and more nervous. Finally, he appeared from behind the curtain.

With the help of the young man, his intern, Dr. Wu asked me questions about my period and the tests I'd had done. Then he held my wrist and took my pulses—the primary diagnostic technique in acupuncture. Reading the pulse of each of the five major subsystems of the body indicates which aren't functioning properly. If I hadn't asked him questions, Dr. Wu probably would not have said much more, but I inquired about the diagnosis and understood it had something to do with the kidney meridian. He then put about three needles in my right ear and a couple in my right hand and told me to lie still and "rerax." The needles were completely painless, but the room was hot and stuffy. I lay there for what seemed like hours, listening to the story of the next patient behind the curtain (chronic headaches), hearing voices of other patients in other rooms (the guy had a real assembly line going here), and trying to "rerax."

To calm myself, I tried some visualization exercises. I imagined myself pregnant, what I would look like and feel like. I looked down at my watermelon belly, cupping my arms around its surprising hardness. I saw myself naked in a full-length mirror admiring my bulges for a change. I envisioned the look of delight on Bill's face when he first felt the kicking. I saw us on a floor somewhere in a Lamaze class huffing and puffing together. I conveniently skipped over childbirth (why ruin a good fantasy?) and then saw myself holding a brand new baby with Bill proudly looking over my shoulder.

After half an hour in fantasyland, however, I was bored and impatient, unable to concentrate and wondering if Dr. Wu had forgotten about me. After another fifteen minutes, he returned, removed the needles, and told me about some herbs he wanted me to take. He wrote the prescription down in Chinese and told me how to prepare them. It sounded very complicated, and I could barely understand a word he said. Before I left I asked the intern to translate the prescription. He also gave me directions to the "pharmacy," a few blocks away on Broadway.

Walking past the Broadway strip joints and into the herb store produced a mild culture shock. I could have just walked off the street in Shanghai. The walls of the high-ceilinged room were lined with huge jars and the floor was covered with barrels, all containing specimens of animal, vegetable, and mineral matter in bizarre shapes and colors. Some were recognizable, like the tiny dried sea horses (Did people actually eat these little guys?), but most were completely unfamiliar. I browsed around, feeling quite conspicuous, until someone spoke to me and I handed him my piece of paper full of Chinese characters. I watched as he weighed out various things and folded them expertly into paper envelopes I hoped I'd be able to refold correctly. In comparison to all the stuff I'd seen there, my particular prescription looked fairly benign—twigs, shavings, dried berries, and pieces of roots. At home, I immediately brewed them up; they tasted foul. I held my breath as I swallowed and wondered what in the hell I was doing.

My first experience with Dr. Wu had not been very pleasant, and he was certainly lacking in the bedside manner category, but I continued to see him for a couple of months. He wanted me to come twice a week. I felt I could only afford once a week, and, I must admit, I did slack off on the herb taking. Maybe that's why his "wizardry" didn't work on me. Or perhaps it was my Western tendency toward impatience. I wanted to get pregnant right away, not spend months awaiting subtle changes in my system. I was not disillusioned with acupuncture, only this particular manifestation, but it added to my growing sense of hopelessness about having a baby.

Throughout this period of waiting for fertility treatment, I continued to contemplate what nonphysical problems might be in the way of my getting pregnant. I knew that some people cure themselves of cancer by changing their ways of thinking and by using visualization techniques that "reprogram" the body to fight the cancer. They visualize armies of white blood cells attacking the cancerous cells and devouring them. They imagine themselves bathed in a white light that heals and strengthens them. I wondered if the same kind of process might increase my fertility.

I began to make my erratic meditations a regular discipline. Often, particularly before, during, and after ovulation, I would lie down, relax, and try to visualize what was going on in my body. I imagined juicy, ripe eggs and robust sperm drawn to each other with incredible intensity. In my imagination, I "talked to" the being who would become our baby. I told her how much we wanted her (we did want a girl), what a fine life she would have with us, and how she would be surrounded with love from so many wonderful people. I told her we were ready for her and asked if there were any reason she didn't want to come through or was postponing her appearance. I must admit I didn't get any clear answers, but I kept on asking. I just kept having the feeling that there was nothing wrong with me or Bill and that there had to be some nonphysical answer to our lack of success.

One day I received a call from my friend Evan. I heard from him a couple of times a year, always out of the blue— literally, for he was always flying around the planet on various mystical missions. Tall, handsome, and enigmatic, Evan is a sort of a New Age renaissance man—a master classical musician, philosopher, entrepreneur, Tai Chi teacher, facilitator of a training program called "Loving Relationships," and a leading proponent and practitioner of a process called "rebirthing."

I had learned about rebirthing years ago through Evan and other friends who had experienced it, and as soon as I spoke to Evan this time, I felt he was appearing, as usual, at just the right moment. Rebirthing is a process of reexperiencing your own birth—not just "remembering" it and talking about it, but physically feeling it and expressing those feelings. It is based on the notion that birth is the primal trauma, a terrifying, wrenching experience of leaving the dark, warm safety of the womb and being convulsed out into the harsh environment of a hospital delivery room. For most people, the rebirthers say, being born was a frightening and painful process that left them with a subconscious impression of pain and negativity, both physical and psychic. Reliving your birth is a form of release—a sort of "primal scream" (though you don't necessarily scream) that allows you to let go of your earliest negative conditioning. In its early days (it was born in California, of course), rebirthing was done in water—a hot tub or a warm pool—to recreate the environment of the womb. It has since evolved to dry land, where the same results are achieved simply by having the person breathe deeply in a particular way.

I told Evan we'd been trying to get pregnant with no luck and asked him if he thought rebirthing might be useful. He said he wasn't going to say it would cure me, but if I had unconscious fears associated with birth, rebirthing could free up that energy and allow me to be more open to giving birth myself. He said he'd be happy to do a session with me. That afternoon we had some herb tea and talked for a while, and then he had me lie down on a pad on the floor and breathe deeply for several minutes. As I inhaled and exhaled slowly, I began thinking about the circumstances of my birth.

It was the height of World War II, and my father was in the Navy on a destroyer in the Atlantic. My mother had brought my sister and brother to live with my grandparents in rural South Carolina, the middle of cotton and tobacco country. I had not been planned for—one of those miracle shore-leave babies who'd ignored both the time of the month and the diaphragm. As I continued to breathe deeply, Evan asked me to go back to the time before I was born. Soon, I stopped thinking and began feeling what it was like to be inside my mother's womb. I had expected it to feel warm and safe, a cozy world all my own. But as I continued to breathe, I did not feel comfortable at all; I felt afraid.

I told Evan I was feeling anxious and fearful, but he had me continue breathing. My breathing grew deeper and faster, and I became more frightened and then panicky. I started crying "Let me out! Let me out of here!" I was writhing around as if struggling with a straitjacket, feeling sheer terror. After a while, I calmed down and just began to cry. As the tide of emotion ebbed, I was able to talk to Evan about what was going on. I interpreted that the anxiety I was feeling was my mother's—her constant fear that my father would not return from the war, that she would end up a war widow with three small children. Perhaps that fear, which I felt along with her, had something to do with my early emergency exit from the womb. Three weeks before her due date, my mother started hemorrhaging severely and had to be rushed forty miles to a city hospital, where I was born by cesarean section.

Evan began asking me questions about what the fear and the birth trauma meant to me, and a rush of feelings came out. "Something is wrong with me.... I wasn't really wanted.... Life is very difficult, and you have to suffer and struggle.... I'm not enough ... I'm not enough." I didn't know where all these thoughts were coming from, but I just let them flow. I cried and cried, and soon the tension seemed to melt out of me.

Then Evan asked me to visualize myself being pregnant and to allow myself to feel all the fears I had about having a baby. First came the fear of miscarriage, of losing a baby so early in its life and so late in my life. What might be very painful for a younger woman could be devastating for me, for what if I never got pregnant again? Then there was the fear of something going wrong in childbirth—of losing the baby at birth and of being unable to cope with the grief. Other fears surfaced. What if I had amniocentesis and found out the baby had Down's syndrome? Would I have an abortion? Would I want to keep the baby? How would Bill and I handle such an issue? What if the baby were born with a major birth defect that had been undetected in pregnancy? How would I respond to an abnormal child?

And then came the fear of childbirth itself, of the pain my friends described as excruciating. How would I manage? Would I freak out, abandon natural childbirth, and beg for anesthesia? What if I had to have a cesarean? And what about my body afterwards? Would I remain fat and dumpy? Would my breasts sag? Would Bill still find me attractive and sexy? My God, with so many fears, no wonder I was having trouble getting pregnant! To complete our session, Evan took me through a meditation process in which I abandoned my fears and embraced my baby. It was a beautiful experience, and by the end of our session I was glowing.

That evening, I curled up with Bill on the couch and told him about my rebirthing experience. I could tell he was somewhat skeptical, but he held me very tenderly and stroked my hair. He said he didn't know if all that I had uncovered had anything to do with getting pregnant, but it was good to be conscious of those fears. He, too, was afraid of many of the same things having to do with my age and its possible effect on the baby. But he had to admit he worried most about what would happen to me physically—whether I would ever recover the shape, slimness, and body tone that he found so attractive. Not that he wouldn't love me, of course, but he hated the thought of me overweight with sagging breasts and belly. He was afraid that I would "never be the same after childbirth" and that he would find me less attractive and sexy.

I knew it was hard for Bill to admit those feelings, so I couldn't jump down his throat as I wanted to. I calmly told him that it scared me to death to hear him say that. "How important is the shape of my body in comparison to having a child?" I found myself being very defensive. "How can you think I'd just let myself go to pot? I've always looked years younger than I am. I've always exercised and been able to lose weight when I wanted to. . . ." Bill backed off, saying it really wasn't that big a deal, and I calmed down. But for days after, as I thought about the rebirthing and all the fears I felt I had been able to let go of, I found I had a new fear, the niggling possibility of a double bind. If I really was infertile, would Bill want to leave me for a younger woman who could give him a baby? Or if I was fertile and did have a baby, would Bill want to leave me for a younger woman with high breasts and no belly?

I knew my fears were unfounded, that Bill and I were so much in love and so committed to our relationship that nothing could come between us. Still, we were feeling the

strain of infertility in our sex life. Now that we had settled
into our ménage à trois with the basal thermometer, our third
partner dictated our lovemaking. I was the one who had
charge of the chart and knew exactly the days of the next
"opportunity." I expected that Bill would also remember
where we were in my cycle, but he was mostly oblivious. The
chart was not etched in his consciousness as it was in mine.
It annoyed me that he took no responsibility in the matter, but
at least he was cooperative in the timing—as long as I reminded him. Basically, the week prior to ovulation was our
celibate period, since Bill was "saving up" his sperm. I imagined the sperm gathering forces in the scrotum like an army
readying for a major offensive. When it was time for the mid-
month onslaught, we would make love no matter what. Neither
exhaustion nor lack of interest could keep us from our duty.
After a couple of perfunctory sessions, we seemed to lose
interest for a while. Then it was almost time for my period
and all that it entailed. Not much space was left for pure,
spontaneous, romantic sex.

Bill made it clear that premeditated lovemaking was a
drag—no longer escape, relief, or rejuvenation, but a source of
frustration and sadness, and ultimately a reminder of failure.
At times he was angry, but usually he didn't direct it at me.
During this period, we were able to talk openly and lovingly
about our predicament and sometimes even laugh at ourselves. We realized that our ability to communicate openly was
one of the benefits of having married late in life. We had both
gained the emotional maturity to avoid anger, accusations,
and blame. We tried to keep perspective and remember that
this was just a phase of our relationship. This, too, would pass.

I still had hope that something, either medical or mystical,
would get me pregnant, but months of trying anything had
brought me no closer to my goal. Obviously, you can't be a
little bit pregnant, so I had no way of knowing if any of my
unorthodox methods were paying off in any way. All I knew

was that I was becoming more and more obsessed, desperately seeking some kind of understanding, some way to make "progress."

Creeping over me was an overwhelming sense of failure. Like most affluent young people of my generation, I had been able to have most of what I wanted in life. Some achievements came easily; some I worked hard for. Some things came to me right when I wanted them; some, like finding the man of my dreams and getting married, took a long time. I had also experienced failure in my life—relationships and jobs that didn't work out, projects I had set in motion but not completed. But in all those circumstances, I could look back and recognize my own responsibility in the matter. I could see what I had done or not done that had contributed to the outcome. Generally, I felt a sense of power and the ability to create my own reality, but here was a situation in which I felt I had no control at all—no power to make happen what I wanted to happen.

Feeling out of control made me both sad and angry. I was being denied one of the most fundamental experiences of being human—procreation. And every day I read about children who were unwanted and mistreated. Why was it so easy for people who didn't want children to have them? Why were monsters who abused children allowed to have them when we were not? Why me? Why us? What was wrong here? Was the problem in our minds or in our bodies?

I knew that all the things I had tried—meditation, acupuncture, psychics, and rebirthing—seemed silly and stupid to many people, yet at least they gave me something to do, some way to combat the helplessness of our situation. As our date with the fertility specialist drew near, I felt a new surge of hope—at last there was something real and scientific we could do. We had the miracles of modern medicine before us, and we would be saved!

Chapter Three

❦

Medicine and Mystery

I had been awaiting the beginning of fertility treatment like a child waiting for Christmas. Surely Dr. B, the specialist, would be our Santa Claus. Our first appointment with him was to be a one-hour consultation in which we would talk about our situation and he would outline possible treatment. When the day finally arrived, we were early and sat nervously in a very large waiting room before being escorted to the doctor's very small office. In such a close setting, it was easy to feel intimate. Plus, we liked the guy right off. He was the opposite of Santa Claus, tall and thin. He was nice-looking, and I could tell from his diplomas that he was about my age (although I always find it hard to believe that doctors and policemen can be my age or younger). On his wall was a knick-knack that he explained was a Japanese fertility symbol—a nice touch. We told him our story, our

frustration over having no real diagnosis, and our anxiety
about moving as quickly as possible because of my age.

His response was reassuring and encouraging. What with
the drugs and technology he had available, he had enough
weapons in his infertility arsenal to overcome age-related problems for a while, so we shouldn't worry about that. He also
told us that his treatment process would not be interminable.
Barring major problems, within a year we could conduct all
the tests and perform all the procedures necessary to get a
result one way or another. Either I'd get pregnant or we would
probably know why not.

First, Dr. B gave us a general overview of the causes of
infertility and told us there were basically four categories of
problems: sperm, ovulation, tubes, and cervix. So far, Bill's
sperm were performing well; it seemed that I was ovulating
regularly; and initial indications were that my tubes were open.
This left the cervical arena, the gate through which sperm must
pass to get to where the action is. Cervical problems are the
easiest to treat, requiring the least invasive as well as the least
expensive treatment. The doctor explained in detail the course
of treatment, which would begin with intrauterine inseminations (IUI) in conjunction with Clomid. We were ideal candidates for IUI, and his results had been fairly good—about
30 percent of his patients got pregnant within six inseminations.

One out of three didn't seem like great odds to me, but
I was excited and happy, certain that we would be among the
lucky ones. We discussed the cost of the treatment, which
would be about $200 per cycle, including the cost of the
Clomid, an ultrasound exam to make sure eggs were present,
and the insemination process. We knew it was unlikely that
our insurance would cover any of this, so we told him we'd
better get the job done fast.

On our way home, Bill and I both felt encouraged. Bill

liked Dr. B and was glad we were at last pursuing a less esoteric treatment process. For me, the only disappointment about the session was that Dr. B wanted to redo some of the tests I had already done with my gynecologist to gather his own evidence and make sure we were on the right track. I had hoped we could start the inseminations right away, but I understood his logic. I made an appointment for a postcoital test a couple of weeks away.

The day of the test was just two days before we were scheduled to leave for a two-week vacation in Hawaii. "Take a vacation" was another popular prescription for getting pregnant, so I had high hopes that all this medical mess would be unnecessary. I imagined calling Dr. B after we returned to tell him aloha and thanks very much but we wouldn't be seeing him after all. And what a perfect place for a little embryo to gestate! I loved Hawaii and was looking forward to sharing it for the first time with Bill.

According to my chart, I was supposed to be ovulating on the day of the test, but the postcoital revealed no mucus at all. Dr. B said he was not really surprised, as one of the side effects of Clomid is to reduce the production of cervical mucus. He wanted me to come back the next day for another test, which I did. It also showed none of the gooey stuff. I was about to write off a vacation-related conception, but on the plane the next day, the mucus was flowing. Ah, my body was just waiting until we got to Hawaii! That night on Maui, we made passionate love to the sound of warm winds blowing through a sugar cane field. As I fell asleep, I prayed to the god of the Hunas that our child would be conceived here in paradise just before my forty-first birthday.

Though I had no bodily symptoms, the feeling that I might be pregnant stayed with me those two weeks on Maui and Kauai. I drifted in the ocean waves imagining an embryo floating in the sea of my belly—life beginning again in my warm inner ocean. On my birthday, we hiked up a stream and discovered a magical spot with crystal pools and a waterfall. Except for the occasional noise of helicopters overhead (called Hawaii's state bird), we had the place to ourselves and celebrated by making love on a flat rock suffused with sunshine. That evening, we climbed to the ruins of one of Kauai's holiest places, the site of the initiation of young Hawaiian kings. Alone again, we sat on rocks that once formed a temple wall and watched the earth turn away from the sun across 300 degrees of ocean horizon. In the inexplicable joy of a perfect birthday, I was certain that we were blessed, that we only had to open ourselves to magic and it would appear.

When we returned home, I still had not started my period and was growing more and more excited. By day 32, I would nervously go to the bathroom every hour or so to make sure it hadn't happened yet. Every twinge in my stomach, every little sensation of slight wetness between my legs sent a shiver of fear through me. As before when I thought I might be pregnant, I didn't tell anyone, though this time I did confide to Bill that I was on a rollercoaster of hope and anxiety—every trip to the bathroom was like a dive that left my heart at the top of the hill. Bill was nervous, too, partly because of the possible pregnancy, but he was also bracing for the storm of disappointment if it were not so. By day 34, I lay awake at night praying that this was it, but the next morning the answer to my prayers was clearly, redly, no.

I moped around for several hours, finally let myself cry, and then got angry. My beautiful Hawaiian babe was not to be. How could I have been so stupid as to hope? I should have just drunk those damn Mai Tais and not worried about it! At four in the afternoon, I called a friend and asked her to meet me at a local bar, where I drank two Mai Tais and a Pina Colada and started feeling better. At home I cried again with Bill and went to bed, still sober—or hopeful—enough to mark my chart with an *X* and look for the date of next month's big chance.

My disappointment and depression would have been heavier save for the prospect of our saving grace, Dr. B and the IUI. But he was not ready to begin the inseminations that month, wanting to do another postcoital to determine if the problem was really with my mucus. I was disappointed and resented having to wait yet another month. I felt silly being upset about it, but at my age each month seemed like a giant step toward the day when it would be too late, when my nest would be empty of eggs and I would be truly barren.

I consoled myself with the fact that I didn't look my age, that I could easily pass for 30, and that I was probably healthier now than in my twenties, thanks to health food and Jane Fonda. I remembered that Sophia Loren had had her first child at 42 and Ursula Andress had had hers at 44. I thrilled at every story I heard of successful births after forty. I didn't worry, as many women do, about having the energy to raise a child in my forties or about handling a teenager in my late fifties. I knew I would continue to be an active and energetic person even in "middle age." Neither I nor my over-40 friends conformed to the images we once had of people our age; we truly looked and felt younger than our parents' generation had. And in this age of modern medicine's magic, we could unwrinkle ourselves, replace hair or dye it, even trade in old organs for new. Motherhood after 40 was no longer a rarity, but unlike face-lifts and transplants, there was indeed a deadline. There is no reversing menopause.

I calmed down about Dr. B and took another postcoital test, which I failed. No mucus present. I was sort of excited —was this a diagnosis? Was Clomid the culprit, assisting ovulation but drying up my cervical mucus? Did this little catch-22 explain why I hadn't gotten pregnant all these months? What a drag! Well, at least we had a specific problem to deal with, a cervical one. Let the inseminations begin!

Intrauterine Insemination, I learned, is a fairly recent medical development. It is distinguished from artificial insemination, which has been around for over a century and is used mostly to inject donor sperm into a woman whose husband's sperm are inadequate. The "artificial" part of the process is that the deposit is made into the vagina without intercourse —with an injection or with a cup placed up against the cervix. The sperm are then captured by the cervical mucus and on their way into the uterus.

In the case of IUI, the sperm are injected directly into the uterus, bypassing the cervix and the need for mucus. Until recently, such a process was unfeasible because the uterus can tolerate only a very tiny amount of semen; larger amounts cause severe and painful cramping. The medical breakthrough leading to IUI was the "washing" of the sperm, a process in which the seminal fluid and the sperm are separated. The ejaculate is diluted with a sterile salt and water solution and then centrifuged until the sperm are highly concentrated into a tiny pellet. The sperm are allowed to incubate for an hour, and the most active, motile ones swim up into the solution above the pellet. This solution of salt, water, and concentrated heavy-duty sperm is used for the insemination. It is introduced into the uterus via a thin plastic tube inserted through the cervix.

Clomid is used to stimulate ovulation, and in order to insure optimal timing for the process, an ultrasound examination is done to make sure there is a mature follicle ready to receive the sperm. The ultrasound exam produces a sonogram, a "sound picture" of the follicle, visible to the naked eye on a TV screen. If an egg is present, you are given an injection of a hormone called human chorionic gonadotropin, or HCG, which will trigger ovulation within twenty-four hours—about the time of the insemination.

Vials, tubes, and shots did not seem like a very romantic way to get pregnant, but Bill and I were long past romance; we wanted results. As the insemination appointment grew closer, we got more and more excited. Dr. B had upped my

Clomid dosage to 150 mg and had scheduled me for a Tuesday morning, day 18 of my cycle, since it seemed I had ovulated on day 19 the last cycle. I told him I was not so sure
about this calculation. The thirty-five-day cycle felt to me like
a one-time aberration, and I usually ovulated on day 16 or 17.
I thought we should do the insemination on that Saturday or
Sunday, but he informed me that he did not usually see patients on weekends.

On the weekend in question, we were invited up to the
Napa Valley with a small "wine group" made up of friends
and friends of friends. Not fancying ourselves connoisseurs,
we were a little nervous about going, but it turned out to be
an unpretentious, fun group. We toured a private winery,
checked into a bed and breakfast, and dined together tasting
various wines throughout dinner and rating them for such
subtleties as "color, nose, and finish." After a few glasses, our
ratings grew rather silly and we dubbed ourselves the "Wha
da Wino" group after someone gave a rating and slurred, "But
wha do I know?" I thoroughly enjoyed what I hoped might
be my last evening as a wino for many months. And even
though we were both somewhat drunk and very tired, we
made love just in case this was indeed the time.

The next morning, I wasn't sure whether it was the wine
or ovulation, but my temperature was up, indicating I had
already ovulated. On Sunday, it was still up, and I was, as we
say, bummed out. We had missed another month, another
minute-hand sweep around the old bio clock. I decided to
get the sonogram anyway, hoping I was wrong.

The ultrasound had been described to me as a painless
process, which it would have been except for the fact that
your bladder must be very, very full to provide the best possible background for the high-frequency sound waves. You are
instructed to drink large quantities of water and not to go to
the bathroom. Lying on the table holding it in for ten for fifteen
minutes was an ordeal, one of the unexpected tortures of

fertility treatment. What was worse, the radiologist confirmed that I had already ovulated; he saw only fluid and no follicles present. Sweet man that he was, he knew my disappointment and didn't charge me, but that was small solace. Dr. B also apologized, swearing he thought we had the right time, but I was angry, certain it was because he didn't want to do the insemination on the weekend.

I complained bitterly to Bill about Dr. B's callousness and began to wonder if we had made the right decision in going with him. I began calling prefertile friends and acquaintances and asking them about other doctors. Nancy had called Dr. B but had never seen him because she didn't like how his receptionist treated her on the phone. A friend of hers had not liked him; she felt he was patronizing. A couple I was acquainted with said they had not had a good rapport with Dr. B, and they resented that he wouldn't perform procedures on weekends, even when the timing was critical. But reports on other doctors weren't great either. It seemed everyone had some complaint about somebody. Evelyn had had a bad experience with Dr. C, whom she had doubts about but kept seeing because she was a woman. It took her months to realize that Dr. C was not really a fertility specialist, and she was very angry about the time lost. Diana found Dr. D to be clinical and insensitive. There were some good reports, too. Beverly raved about Dr. E and how comfortable she felt with him, claiming he was the best in the area. But of course I'd have to wait another few months if I wanted to see him.

Everyone who had been through the fertility grind told me how important it was to have a doctor you liked and whom you trusted to know what he was doing. I could see that for me, as for many other women, the fertility doctor would become the second most important man in my life. Though I hoped the relationship would be short-lived, I knew it could last for years—perhaps with two, three, or more different doctors—and was fraught with all the dangers of intense relationships: resentment over their power, need for emotional support, fear of rejection, hurt and anger over unmet expectations.

As I contemplated the doctor–patient relationship, I also began to consider the other side of the relationship, the pressure on the specialist to be a miracle worker and to respond sensitively to women in various degrees and stages of emotional distress. It must be incredibly draining to bear such responsibility day after day and to suffer the failures so frequent in this field. I also realized that I couldn't just make Dr. B my saviour or my scapegoat; I had to take responsibility for my own situation and educate myself so that I could interact knowledgeably with medical professionals.

From my friend Lana I learned about RESOLVE, a national organization for infertile couples. I hadn't heard of the group, but I liked the name: It could connote one's resolve to have a baby no matter what, or to find a resolution if the "no matter what" didn't work. Lana and her husband Ron had participated in a RESOLVE support group, five or six couples and a facilitator who met regularly to discuss the medical, emotional, interpersonal, and financial issues of infertility. They had found the group really valuable but were no longer involved, since they had had their baby. The week after the abortive IUI attempt, Lana called to tell me about a day-long conference sponsored by RESOLVE. It would address the medical and emotional aspects of infertility, and one of the workshops was to be led by Dr. B on intrauterine insemination. I called and signed up right away.

I wanted very much for Bill to go with me to the conference, but I knew that baby making was not really his priority now. His construction business was growing from a two-man operation to a real company with several employees. He had two major projects under way and was working at his limit, including nights and weekends. He felt that if we were going to have a child, he needed to focus on building a financial base for our family. Although running a business was new for him, he was as determined about it as I was about getting pregnant. I forgave him the lack of devotion to my cause, knowing we were both working for the same thing—a family.

The morning of the conference I drove alone to Palo Alto, over an hour's drive on a foggy morning, feeling very sad that it had come to this. I was now part of a group formed around a dysfunction, sort of like Alcoholics Anonymous. I wondered if we would each stand up at the workshop and say, "My name is Mary, and I am infertile...."

Actually, it wasn't so bad. The group was large, made up mostly of women in their thirties and early forties and a few brave husbands. The men might not have come had they known they would come under mild attack. One of the topics of the morning session was how infertility affects relationships, and it was pretty apparent that the largely female audience felt the suffering of the situation was primarily theirs to bear. There were snickers of agreement when one of the panelists mentioned the difficulty in getting men to talk about the problem, especially facing the possibility that the problem might be theirs. But a male panelist took their part, talking about the difficulty of performing on demand and about the feelings of inadequacy that inevitably result from this most basic expression of male ego. Members of the audience shared their personal experiences—marriages almost breaking up, long periods of no communication, financial stress, and fights over differing levels of commitment to treatment.

I knew Bill and I were not equally committed to having a baby, but we had accepted each other's position and didn't fight about it. I began to feel very grateful that we had not yet encountered this array of problems. Still, we were only in our second year of trying and our first month of treatment. Some of these couples had been at it for several years. Was this the picture of things to come?

At coffee breaks, I found myself keeping somewhat apart

from people, overhearing conversations about this and that doctor, this and that treatment, how someone finally had twins and someone else got a divorce. I'm not sure why I kept myself on the fringes, eating lunch alone on the grass while everyone else talked Pergonal and in vitro. Perhaps it was because this was a sorority I did not really want to belong to. Besides, I would not be around for long—the insemination next week would save me from pledging.

In the afternoon seminar, Dr. B was at his most charming describing the delicacies of IUI. Although I already knew much of what he talked about, I was completely fascinated with the details of how the clomiphene works to foster ovulation, how it affects the mucus, how the HCG shot triggers ovulation, and how the seminal fluid is "washed" to become a supersperm solution. In just a few days, I would be living this microscopic drama, and to me it took on epic significance. I found myself mellowing toward Dr. B, appreciating his intelligence, articulateness, and sense of humor. I decided to forget about last month's disappointment and look ahead to a successful future.

At the end of the seminar, we discussed the bitter topic of insurance coverage for infertility treatment. With a very few exceptions, health insurance carriers will not pay for fertility procedures, unless you can disguise them in some way. Because infertility is viewed as a "minority" problem (middle-class women), insurance companies have been able to stonewall, simply refusing to treat it like any other medical condition. How is failure of the reproductive system different from failure of the heart or lungs? Dr. B grew indignantly eloquent about how insurance will pay for triple bypass heart surgery for a man who has drunk alcohol, smoked cigarettes, not exercised, and eaten a high-fat diet all his life, but it will not pay for a woman to fulfill her most fundamental physical need—to have a baby. Everyone in the audience agreed something was wrong here.

Another seminar I attended, an overview of the infertility treatment process, addressed some of the economic issues of infertility. Participants in the group told of spending tens of thousands of dollars on various tests, medications, and surgeries. Some reported that they were able to get their insurance to cover part of the costs, but even paying 20 percent was strapping them. Others told how to disguise certain procedures so they wouldn't look fertility-related. There were a few sad stories of people who thought they had coverage but found out after the fact that the insurance company wouldn't pay. I thought of the hundreds of thousands, perhaps millions, of couples who simply could not afford the amount of money we were talking about. Looking around the room, it seemed pretty obvious that the couples here were predominantly white upper middle class, the fortunate few who could afford to contemplate such expenditures. Surely infertility wasn't confined to the affluent, but treatment seemed to be.

During the seminar, there was much discussion of the two high-tech solutions to infertility, in vitro fertilization, IVF for short—and gammete intrafallopian transfer—or GIFT. This was the first time I had heard so much about these two operations. It was somewhat confusing at first, but I came to understand what the two procedures are and how they differ. Both involve the use of fertility drugs to stimulate ovulation, retrieval of one or more eggs through surgery or ultrasound technique, and the mixing of sperm and eggs outside the body. In IVF, which bypasses the fallopian tubes entirely, fertilization takes place in a laboratory dish. The embryos (usually more than one) are incubated for a few days and then transferred into the woman's uterus, where, you hope, one will implant and begin a successful pregnancy. In the GIFT procedure, one open tube is needed so the sperm and egg mixture can be injected directly into it and fertilization can then take place in the body's natural environment.

Both of these procedures are highly invasive, physically

and emotionally demanding, and very expensive. What's worse, the odds are not good. For a cost of $5000 to $8000, IVF promises a pregnancy rate of 5 to 20 percent per cycle. At $3000 to $6000, GIFT is somewhat better, with a success rate of 10 to 25 percent per cycle. Very few insurance companies will cover either procedure, although some will cover the cost of the Pergonal injections—about $750 to $1500.

These high-tech solutions would, I fervently hoped, never be necessary for us. I could not imagine how we would afford them. But it was not just the money; it was the emotional cost that seemed the highest. The infertility veterans I was encountering here did seem like they had been through a war. They were well versed in the weapons and the strategies, able to discuss the variables and technicalities as if they were medical students. They had a camaraderie with the doctors and many of the other participants, and they seemed weary and sad. There had been a few laughs during the day, but for me the tone of this conference had been fairly grim, and I left feeling somewhat depressed. I did feel comforted that there were a lot of other people going through the same thing I was. I just prayed I would not have to go as far as they had.

It was just a few days later that I had my first intrauterine insemination. I endured the ultrasound water torture, and this time there were follicles, two of them, picked up by the sound waves. The radiologist positioned the monitor screen so I could see them—one good-sized, the other a little smaller. He measured them with some instrument and then called Dr. B's office to confirm we had eggs. As I experienced the profound pleasure of letting go of all that water, I rubbed my belly and said, "Get ready, girls. Tomorrow is your big day."

The next morning, Bill preferred to be alone for the "specimen gathering," which was fine with me since he had to leave early for work. He left the white plastic cup on the kitchen table, and when I looked inside, I was a little nervous. It seemed like there was only about a teaspoon of seminal fluid in there—would it be enough? Were there really billions and billions of little beings in there? Was one of them to become our offspring? I wasn't quite sure what to do with the little white cup on the drive into the city—should I keep it warm or cool, put it in my purse or between my legs? What if it somehow spilled out through the top? I drove very carefully, as if my passenger were a sensitive time bomb.

No one was in Dr. B's office when I arrived, but there were three brown bags with names on them sitting outside the door. I assumed they had little white cups inside, and I was horrified. People could actually drop the stuff off like that, leaving them there like little orphans on a doorstep! I could never do such a thing! I waited for Dr. B's assistant, delivered the goods in hand, and then tried to figure out what to do with myself for the next three hours. It was too early to go shopping. I killed time at a local cafe, walked around, and looked at clothes I knew I could not afford to buy.

Even though Bill's presence was not necessary, I wanted him to be there for the conception of his child and he agreed to join me. I waited anxiously for him in the waiting room, prepared to be very upset if he didn't show up. He was already half an hour late. When he rushed in, out of breath, he grabbed me and apologized. He'd been nervous all morning, he said, and had left work with just enough time to get there. But he had had to stop for gas so he wouldn't run out on the Golden Gate Bridge and then had gotten lost and couldn't find a parking place. He'd run several blocks, afraid he'd missed it. We hugged and almost cried together. Luckily, the doctor was running behind.

A few minutes later, Dr. B invited us into the tiny lab room for a look at the sperm (I guess there was plenty if he could show some off to us), and Bill got quite a kick out of it. We were nervous and joking, Bill telling the doctor that he was starting to have "little white cup fantasies." Dressed in the red flowered Chinese robe Dr. B provided, I climbed into the stirrups with Bill by my side. Getting sperm into my uterus was not a rapturous experience. The speculum was cold, my vagina was tight, and fitting the tube into the cervical opening was downright painful. It took about a minute but seemed like five. Dr. B kept telling me to relax; I kept squeezing Bill's hand white and trying not to yell. How romantic can you get?

When the deed was done and the doctor had left with instructions to lie still for five minutes or so, Bill and I embraced and kissed, trying to create some semblance of love-making in this bizarre process. As I lay on the table, he held me close and talked about how we'd be together like this nine months from now, huffing and puffing our way through childbirth. He said he felt my body was "a magical temple of birth," and stroked my belly lovingly. We both felt our love so strongly at that moment, how could it not incorporate itself into our child?

Bill had to get back to work, and I drove home alone, once again envisioning the momentous events I hoped were going on inside of me. At home, I lay quietly on the couch for an hour listening to soothing music, meditating on cell division, and praying that I would be delivered into the land of the fertile.

A few days later I had a blood test to determine the level of progesterone in my blood, and the doctor said it was "sky-high." I had definitely had a good ovulation, and my hopes soared. One morning I awoke from a wonderful dream. Right in front of my face had appeared the face of a smiling baby, a beautiful baby who looked like us! I was thrilled, thinking our child-to-be had checked in to say hello. I kept the image of that face before me and told all my friends about it. So sure was I of that sign that I could hardly believe it when my period started. I went to bed and cried.

Back on the roller coaster, we got ourselves up for another try a month later. Bill came with me again, and we had the same intense experience of love but not the same measure of hope. We were almost afraid to be hopeful once again. By the time we got to insemination number three, we were worried and unenthusiastic. I found myself dropping off the jar of orphan sperm at the door, hurrying to make a meeting. Bill begged off from joining me because of problems on the job, and I went back to work after five wistfully hopeful minutes on the table. All the meditation and prayer were seeming a little silly by now, but I tried to be positive. Two weeks later the results were negative.

During that summer of unsuccessful inseminations, I felt that everything else in my life, particularly my career, was on hold. Living in prefertile limbo, I found myself facing what turned out to be an old-fashioned identity crisis. For several years, I had been working as a free-lance writer and media producer, putting together film, video, and multi-image projects for corporate and educational clients. I had just finished working as a writer and researcher on a documentary for PBS and was hoping to do more of the same, perhaps as a producer. But clearly, my heart wasn't in it. The projects I had in mind languished right there, as I seemed able to mobilize energy only around the idea of becoming a mother. It was a strange new world for me. I had always been ambitious, a "go-getter," but now all I wanted to get was pregnant.

Perhaps as a result, perhaps by coincidence, my work started drying up. I had always experienced the free-lance life as drought and monsoon, but usually the pattern changed rather quickly. This time, the drought dragged on through the summer. Just when I could have used a lot of diversion, I found myself with time on my hands and very little desire to make anything happen. If I got a big project going, would the stress and pressure interfere with getting pregnant? What if I did get pregnant? Would I just drop the project? Would I want to continue to work with a new baby? I talked to my prefertile friends about it and found they had felt the same way. Beverly had cut back on the number of patients she was seeing, hoping to remove some "stress" from her life. Diana had refused a promotion at work and was even considering taking another job that would give her better health insurance. Almost everyone else felt that their ambition had dried up, that they didn't have the energy to drive themselves through both fertility treatment and career mobility. That I was not alone in my feelings didn't help much. I began to wonder if my feelings weren't just an excuse for being lazy or afraid to pursue new career goals.

Except for the monthly flurry of fertility treatment, I had few demands on me from the outside, but a lot of "should" demands from myself: I should be writing. I should be taking writing courses. I should be looking harder for free-lance jobs. I should put together a proposal for the documentary I've been thinking about. I should get a "real job," a nine-to-five, paying job, with health insurance. I should do all those little things I said I would do when I had time, like putting our photos in albums or transferring my hodgepodge folder of recipes to neat 5×7 cards. I should get more involved in the issues I care about—ending world hunger and the nuclear arms race. I should become a Big Sister to some needy child or volunteer at some community agency. Day after day, I should-ed myself into near paralysis.

Meanwhile, Bill's focus remained on building his company. He continued to work days, nights, and weekends trying to keep on top of things. I resented that he had little time to spend with me or to fulfill my free-time fantasies of going backpacking in the Sierra and visiting Mendocino and Big Sur. He resented that I wasn't working and that I was spending my time moping around the house. We both felt the added pressure of no income on my part at a time when the inseminations were adding $250 to our monthly expenses.

During the first month of the drought, I did manage to write an article about what we had been going through in our first year and a half of waiting for baby. I sent the article to a newspaper syndicate but got no response for over a month.

With the encouragement of a friend, I persevered and sent inquiries to a dozen women's magazines. I received as many rejections, nice and impersonal: "The article doesn't meet our needs at this time." I started feeling infertile as a writer as well.

The rejections helped cement my state of depression: I was a failure as a writer, and I was a failure as a woman. I used the New Age philosophy that says we each create our own reality to blame myself for creating a childless one. My mother offered encouragement and advice, suggesting that I take in a foster child for a while—"to see what it's like to have a child." I was annoyed. I didn't need to see what it was like, I needed my own baby. I felt so drained, I had no energy for a problem child, and Bill certainly didn't.

He would leave for work at 6:00 in the morning and come home at night exhausted. I'd feed him dinner (grocery shopping and cooking gourmet meals were a good diversion, but they had consequences in the weight category), and he'd be back at work for a few hours until bedtime. He was emotionally supportive, trying to help me motivate myself, but he just couldn't spend more time with me at this crucial time of building his business. After a particularly gruesome week of wandering around the house wondering what to do, I decided I needed to see a therapist. My friend Katherine recommended Sharon, an older woman whom I met with and liked right away.

Long-haired and somewhat Bohemian-looking, Sharon was the type Woody Allen would cast as a therapist. She was a New Age type who drew upon spiritual as well as emotional therapy processes. In our first couple of sessions, I kept trying to analyze what was going on with me, but Sharon encouraged me to stop talking and just let myself cry. Finally, I let myself indulge in self-pity, feeling sorry for myself for not having a baby, for not having work, and for feeling hopeless and helpless on both counts.

Tearfully, I began to delve into feelings of powerlessness and inferiority. What was wrong with me? Then I wallowed in the mud of guilt and self-reprobation: It was all those years of being single and sexually active. I was a bad girl, and now I was being punished. I should have settled down in my twenties. I shouldn't have smoked pot. I didn't deserve to be with Bill; he should find someone younger who could give him children years from now when he was totally ready. If only we'd met earlier. . . . If only I weren't like this. . . . If only. . . .

All my life, in all the therapy I had done over the years, the problem boiled down to the fact that I wasn't enough. I hadn't done enough, couldn't do enough, couldn't be enough to have what I wanted in life. My infertility confirmed this diagnosis.

Experiencing and expressing all these pent-up emotions brought me to a breakthrough of sorts. In our third session, while talking about how bad I felt about not working, I realized that throughout my life, my self-esteem had always been based on what I did—on my work and what I accomplished. Not being able to "accomplish" having a baby was a direct attack on my self-worth. But if I were indeed to become a mother, I would face another challenge. Would I consider changing diapers and taking care of baby a worthy accomplishment? Would it fulfill my perception of myself as a modern superwoman? Or would I find myself dissatisfied after a few months, ready to get an au pair and go back to work in the real world?

I realized that if I was to be truly happy as a mother, I needed to find another source of self-esteem. I needed to love myself for who I was as well as for what I did. To be happy in the role of nurturer, I needed to learn how to be more receptive, to *be* as well as to *do*. Perhaps my lack of receptivity was what was psychically blocking pregnancy. Sharon suggested I explore more of the feminine aspect of myself, that I stop trying to "push through" everything and rather learn to yield, to accept, and to cultivate, God forbid, *patience*.

Just *being* is not as easy as it sounds. Sharon suggested that I start by meditating. I had practiced meditation for a number of years, but that was several years ago, and whatever ability to quiet the mind I had gained in the laid-back seventies had drained away in the get-it-all-now eighties. Once a day, I dutifully sat quietly while my mind raged on noisily, running over and over its list of complaints and shoulds. At times I would try to concentrate on getting pregnant, visualizing myself fat and happy and then giving birth. But Sharon cautioned me about trying to "do" things with meditation. I was falling into the old pattern of trying to make something happen rather than just being receptive.

During one session when I was particularly desolate, Sharon asked to me write a list of all the things I would do if I had all the money I wanted and had already achieved all the things I wanted to accomplish in life. It was difficult at first to think about just what I wanted to do rather than what I should do. I felt guilty writing down things like "Go shopping and buy expensive clothes and jewelry" and "Travel around the world and meet all the people I'd like to know." Clearly, these weren't options now, but there were a surprising number of things on my list that I actually could do right then and there. "Be a really good tennis player": I found a partner and started taking lessons. "Grow a fabulous flower garden": I planted a small plot with summer flowers. "Write regular commentaries on various subjects for the newspapers and TV": I wrote a couple of commentaries and sent them to National Public Radio's "All Things Considered." "Lie in the sun and swim in warm water": I gave myself permission to hang out at our neighborhood pool.

All the time I was practicing *being*, my mind chattered to me about how I was just being lazy and self-indulgent and how gardening and meditation had nothing to do with getting pregnant. I would still try to "program" myself for pregnancy. As I swam laps in the pool, I would recite the mantra in my mind, "I am ready to be pregnant and deliver a healthy baby." Although I still desperately wanted the inseminations to work,

I found myself relaxing a little about it all. In one conversation with Sharon, I realized that I had spent so many years being unhappy because I didn't have a man in my life. Now I had the man, but I was making myself unhappy about not having a child. Did I really want to spend more of my life unhappy and dissatisfied?

As I began to give myself more permission to just be with myself and pursue activities I enjoyed without feeling guilty, I started to feel a new peace in my life. Bill and a number of my friends commented that I seemed to have changed, that I was happier and more relaxed. Bill was even a little jealous and tried to make more time to spend with me.

During my *being* period, I tried to imagine what it would be like to live the rest of my life without children, being, as they say, "childfree." I thought a lot about our friends Kurt and Ingrid, who had done some very wise real estate investing in the seventies and were reaping the benefits now. Early in their marriage, they had agreed they would not have children, and now, in their forties, they spent their time and money transforming their house and garden into a magical little estate and traveling several times a year. They flew first class to Europe to ski, spent a month in the South Seas, took the Queen Elizabeth II across the Atlantic, and tripped off whenever they pleased to Mexico or Hawaii. Clearly, they weren't saving for anyone's college education.

There must be some kind of gene some people have that says "You've got to have children." As I've talked to other people—mostly women—I've found almost no one who was really torn or confused about the issue. You either want them or you don't, and women seem to be pretty clear about which it is by their mid-thirties. The freedom and affluence of Kurt and Ingrid's lifestyle was definitely appealing, but try as I might to imagine ourselves in their shoes, I couldn't. I simply could not imagine a life without children, and I knew that even if we had to go to Timbuktu to get one, I was going to raise at least one child.

My determination to have children made me impatient with fertility treatment, and I began to bug Dr. B with questions about IUI. Why wasn't it working? I wanted him to give me an answer, but he could only shrug, raise his eyebrows, and shake his head. We looked like perfect candidates for this procedure, he kept saying, and he couldn't say why it hadn't worked. What could be wrong, of course, was something with my tubes. Since the hysterosalpingogram (the blue dye test) was not conclusive and could not rule out endometriosis, we could be wasting our time with the IUI. Since the next window of opportunity coincided with Dr. B's month-long vacation, I decided to go ahead and have a laparoscopy as soon as possible.

A laparoscopy is performed to get a direct view of the tubes, ovaries, and uterus to determine if there are abnormalities affecting fertility. It is a fairly simple operation, usually performed on an outpatient basis, so that you are in and out of the hospital on the same day. The laparoscope, a thin tube of a microscope, is inserted through an incision at the navel. If adhesions are found, regular surgery or laser surgery can be performed immediately, making it possible to clear the tubes and remove any endometriosis without another operation.

For my laparoscopy, I returned to Dr. A, my gynecologist, who was reputed to be an expert at laser surgery should such be necessary. He had done outpatient surgery on me a few years before, for an inflamed gland in my vagina, and I felt comforted that I was in his hands. I reported to Same Day Surgery very early on a cold, foggy morning. Bill dropped me off and would return later in the day to pick me up. I signed what seemed like dozens of forms, put on the obligatory green gown, and talked to a nice anesthesiologist. He gave me a shot of Demerol to relax me, and when Dr. A came by to see how I was doing, I said, "We've got to stop meeting like this." By the time I was wheeled into the operating room, I was pretty loopy and started asking him all the questions I had had on my mind as his patient for all these years: "Why aren't you married?" "Do you have a girlfriend?" "Are you living together?" "When are you going to get married?" He was polite but embarrassed, and the nurses were giggling. Lucky for us both, the sodium pentothal sent me into never-never land by the count of two.

When I came to in the recovery room, I was disoriented, to say the least. My mind was filled with strange images I couldn't seem to focus into a coherent picture. When the nurse came over to ask me how I was, I kept saying over and over, "Weird thoughts, weird thoughts." They were clearly worried about me. At some point, Dr. A came in to tell me the results of the operation. I recognized him, and we seemed to have a normal conversation, but after he was gone, I couldn't remember anything he said. I was taken back to the Same Day Surgery waiting room and hung around in a big reclining chair feeling wretched. The anesthesia had made me quite nauseous, and I was throwing up every ten or fifteen minutes, unable to keep down soda crackers or even water. Finally, Bill came to take me home and asked anxiously about what the doctor had found. I said I couldn't remember and didn't care. Get me to bed....

It wasn't until the next morning that I reached Dr. A by phone to find out the results. He had found a few adhesions—"no big deal"—and no sign of endometriosis. But he had found a small ovarian cyst, which he had removed. Unfortunately, the cyst probably had had no effect on my ovary and ovulation process, so I couldn't really count it as a diagnosis for infertility. Again, I didn't know whether to be glad or sad. The fact that everything looked good, that my tubes were open and my ovaries looked fine, should have been encouraging. But I was disappointed. I wanted a reason, a diagnosis, something to treat, something to do something about! Now it seemed like we were back at square one.

Feeling sad and shaky, I lay in bed contemplating the stitches in my navel and the future of our efforts to make a baby through the miracles of modern medicine. Not a pretty picture. So far, we had spent more than $3000 in our efforts to make a baby. Dr. B would do three more inseminations at about $250 each. If one of them didn't work, the next logical step would be to try the drug Pergonal, which could cost up to $1500 per cycle. If that didn't work, we'd be faced with trying IVF or GIFT, which meant thousands more dollars out of pocket. And the odds—one in five or less—were not the kind a reasonable person would bet money on.

My faith that technology would save us was wearing thin. Bill, too, was discouraged. He suggested we just give up on it for a year or so; then he wouldn't feel he had to work so hard. We could spend more time together, and when we did start up again, he would be more enthusiastic and supportive. I reminded him that in a few months I would turn 42. I felt strongly that we didn't have a couple of years to wait.

When Dr. B returned from vacation, I reviewed our situation with him. Bill had good sperm. I ovulated and had open tubes. On at least three occasions, sperm and egg had been put in close proximity to each other. Why were we still waiting for baby? He shrugged and said that medical understanding of fertility was still in its infancy, that we just hadn't figured out all the factors and variables governing reproduction. Who knew what tiny, undetectable, possibly simple problem could be responsible? What he was doing, he said, was as much art as science. For the first time, I sensed some of his discouragement about the two-thirds of his patients he could not help. In that moment I felt we both shared a resigned respect for the mysteries of the creation of life.

"God giveth and God taketh away," came into my mind as I pondered those mysteries. Still I prayed that God or medicine or mystery would make me a baby, that I would yet become fruitful and multiply.

Chapter Four

❦

Facing Failure, Finding Resolution

*T*he laparoscopy marked the beginning of our third year of Trying. For one cycle after the operation, we took a break from the grind of treatment—no thermometers, white cups, or stirrups for a month. It was a blessed relief, but I still made sure we made love mid-month and lived in mild hope for a couple of weeks that we would do it "naturally." I grew more worried after a postoperative checkup by Dr. A. I was questioning him further about the laparoscopy, and he said that one thing it revealed was that I seemed to be running low on eggs. He said this very casually, but I freaked out. I had started my period at a very early age—I had just turned 11; did this mean I was headed for an early menopause? When I talked to Dr. B about it, he played it down, annoyed at his colleague for mentioning it, but I began to feel even more anxious and impatient.

At about this time, the article I had written months before,

"Waiting for Baby," was finally accepted for publication by the *San Francisco Chronicle*. It appeared as the lead article in the "People" section, nearly two pages with an awful illustration (a forlorn-looking woman) and an okay picture of me and Bill. "Great!" Bill joked, "Now the entire Bay Area knows I can't get my wife pregnant." Actually, he found the publicity kind of fun. It opened up new areas of conversation with people, and he was able to joke about it.

I was surprised and pleased by the response the article generated. For a few weeks after it appeared, I received dozens of letters and telephone calls from other prefertiles, ex-infertiles, adoptive mothers, and other well-meaning people offering advice ranging from interesting to outrageous. One ex-infertile counseled us never to lose hope, that "every penny you spend and every tear of frustration you shed will be worth it when you hold that baby in your arms!" A chiropractor sent us a long letter telling the story of a prefertile patient of his who got pregnant after he treated her lower back area. He believed that adjusting her spine and removing pressure on the nerves in the lower back—the area that supplies the sex organs, uterus, bladder, and knees—had enabled her body to function as it should. He enclosed a chart of the effects of spinal misalignments and information about "vertebral subluxation"—the spine out of place.

Another letter warned us that we might have "too good of a sex life," claiming that vaginal orgasms after ovulation cause the uterus to contract, aborting an embryonic conception and bringing on menstruation. The writer, a woman, suggested that I have only clitoral orgasms in order to get pregnant and have only clitoral orgasms during pregnancy. She offered to send me her book on this subject.

Then there was a six-page letter from a sweet Christian astrologer who advised me to talk to God and to surrender the desire to Him. She then told me I would conceive, during a water sign—good aspects particularly when Venus was in

Scorpio. Another Christian was not so sweet, suggesting this was God's judgment and that I should not go to psychics and should not try to have a baby "in a not-normal way."

Another recommendation from several folks was that we join a support group for infertile couples sponsored by RE-SOLVE. Bill didn't feel we needed group support, but I felt it couldn't hurt to check it out. Within a couple of weeks, we were contacted about a new group starting up in our area, and Bill agreed to go to at least one meeting.

We gathered in a small house in Sausalito. Waiting for everyone to arrive, I ate too many chocolate chip cookies and examined all the photos on the refrigerator door and around the house. I knew these kids must have been adopted, since our hostess, the RESOLVE leader, was supposedly infertile. I searched for the lack of resemblance, but it was hard to tell. When we got under way, there were four couples and a woman who was there without her partner. Our leader, Camile, told her story first, a complex saga of various fertility problems and treatment, miscarriages, adoption, and then a successful pregnancy that was spent mostly in bed. She was articulate and obviously knowledgeable, having led these groups for several years. Then we went around the room telling about our experiences.

Not surprisingly, it was the woman in each couple who spoke first, sometimes tearfully, reciting the familiar litany of tests, hopes, treatments, and disappointments. The husband would then follow up with his perspective. Though the comments by the men were shorter and not so emotional, it was clear that they were as engaged in this process as their wives, just a little less comfortable talking about it. All the stories were similar—we were all in our second or third year of Trying, except for the single woman, who had had a child in an earlier marriage and was now unable to conceive in a new relationship with a younger man. Two couples were in their late twenties; the rest of us, in our late thirties and early forties. One couple had tubal problems and had had a series of operations. Another couple was being treated for a low sperm count. The others, like us, did not yet have a diagnosis and were as frustrated as we were.

When we had all talked and everyone was clearly pretty depressed, Camile, our facilitator, talked at length about the emotional consequences of infertility, and we shook our heads in agreement. No, it's not fair. Yes, it's difficult to face up to the problem and get help. No, you can't expect your friends and family to know how to react sensitively. Yes, it's normal to resent your fertile friends and family and to hate going to family gatherings and baby showers. Yes, medical treatment is expensive and time-consuming and emotionally demanding. No, you're not crazy for feeling crazed most of the time. No, it's not fair. It's definitely not fair. . . .

Most of the discussion that evening focused on how we handled infertility in our lives, and it was apparent that despite the supposed enlightenment of our day, the stigma of the barren woman remains imprinted on our psyches like a scarlet letter. Even though it may be the man who has the fertility problem, it is generally the woman who is considered to be infertile. There are no visible signs of infertility, male or female, but by its absence the pregnant belly condemns the woman rather than her partner. Unable to fulfill our biological destiny, women feel shame and guilt. What did I do to deserve this? Why me?

I guess that's why the women in the group did most of the talking. But, finally, one of the men, who had a low sperm count with low motility, started sharing the agonies of "feeling like less than a man." He, too, felt ashamed and inadequate, afraid that he might even become impotent. He was afraid to tell his male friends and even admitted that he would hint to them that the problem lay with his wife. His admission was a brave one, and his wife hugged him forgivingly. The group seemed more open now, and the other men started talking more. Everyone said they would return in a couple of weeks.

Driving home from the meeting, Bill was very quiet. Finally, he spoke emphatically: "I never want us to become that obsessed with having a baby." He almost sounded angry. "I don't want you to be embarrassed and ashamed, and I don't want to go through years of this soul searching. I'm just not willing to have our life defined by being infertile, to have it be the central fact of our lives. If you really want to have children, then we had better start talking seriously about adoption."

In fact, I had already been talking about adoption with Sharon, my therapist. She was an adoptive mother and felt it was the best decision she had ever made. From the moment her daughter came to her, she told me, she never thought once that she wasn't "hers." I believed her and knew that adoption might be the only way we could have a child, but I still didn't want to face it. A baby from our gene pool would undoubtedly be beautiful, intelligent, graceful, and athletic. Who knew what we'd get from a pair of people we didn't even know? How could anyone else's baby measure up?

But in response to Bill's adamant plea, I began to look at my preconceptions about adoption and to think about mothering "someone else's child." What came to the surface were the basic societal prejudices about adoption—that it was "settling for second best," that adoptive children would somehow be handicapped from having lost contact with their blood parents, that "being adopted" would be an issue for both parents and child throughout life, and that someday the child would want to find his or her "real parents," a process that would be difficult and painful for everyone involved. I knew these stereotypic thoughts were not necessarily true, but that they arose so easily in my thinking indicated their prevalence in our culture.

As Bill and I began to talk about adoption, he said that if we were going to pursue it, he would prefer foreign adoption, giving a home to a child from a poor country who was really needy. He said he wanted to express his commitment to a One World philosophy by creating his own little melting pot family. It was not just a political statement, however. He liked the idea of having an exotic-looking child rather than a "boring WASP." I was somewhat surprised by his attitude and started trying to adjust to the idea of a child who did not look anything like either of us. I tried to fantasize about where our baby would come from, and my thoughts drifted off to Nepal and Thailand.

One of my fondest memories was a trip I had made to Nepal ten years ago. I loved the country—its spectacular scenery, breathtaking mountains, and ancient culture. But I especially loved the people, who were beautiful, warm, and friendly. On the streets and walking through villages, I met lots of Nepali kids, who loved to tag along with Americans. Some of them were orphans who begged me to take them home with me. And there was one in particular I did want to take home, a dark-eyed beauty with a smile the size of Everest. That smile always haunted me.

On the flight back to the States, my plane stopped in Bangkok, where a young American army officer and his wife got on accompanied by five Thai children ranging in age from 2 months to 3 years. As I marveled at the entourage, the stewardess told me that the couple was adopting them all. Astounded at their magnanimity (or was it their craziness?), I approached the harried young mother and asked if I could help her out. Looking like she was about to burst into tears, she thanked me profusely and handed me the 2-month-old and a bottle of formula. For the next few hours, I played mom to this dark-haired bundle, holding him, feeding him, and falling in love with his round face and almond eyes. As it turned out, the overwhelmed young couple was just accompanying the children to the States to join other adoptive parents. They had to keep up the front of being parents to avoid problems with the Thais, who were not happy about kids being taken from their country.

Those few hours with the Thai baby had stayed with me, and he began to inhabit my adoption fantasies, along with Cambodian refugees and my Nepali orphan. I even bought a book about foreign adoption, but I got discouraged as I read it. The couple in the book had ended up adopting two babies, one Chinese and one Colombian, but not without what seemed like a gargantuan struggle. Was it always this difficult? Camile, from RESOLVE, referred me to Cheryl, who was trying to adopt a baby from Honduras, and her story was even more depressing.

According to Cheryl, foreign adoption "is not for the weak of heart." After years of infertility, an ectopic pregnancy that left her with only one tube, and two unsuccessful in vitro attempts, she and her husband, Richard, had decided to adopt. Richard was British, they both had traveled the world, and Cheryl had lived for four years in Central America. They felt like "world citizens" and wanted to give a home to a child from another country, one who would otherwise grow up in an orphanage like the ones Cheryl had worked in in Guatemala. The fact that Cheryl spoke fluent Spanish would, they thought, surely facilitate the process.

With the help of a local adoption service specializing in international adoptions, Cheryl and Richard began making contacts in South America, first in Chile, then in Brazil. But in each case, local political conditions intervened—not an uncommon occurrence. Finally, they found a lawyer who knew of a baby just born in Honduras. The mother was an unmarried domestic servant who could not afford to keep her son. Cheryl and Richard would need to pay for foster care, about $150 a month, and the lawyer's fee of $4000.

When they agreed to take the baby, they had no idea that

the ensuing adoption process would entail three trips to Honduras and nine months in the maddening maze of a Central American bureaucracy. It would have been longer had Cheryl not camped on an administrator's doorstep and begged for an earlier appointment. They were able to have Antonio with them in their hotel while they were there, but they had to return him to the foster home each time they left. It was so painful to leave him, especially when they had no idea how long it would be before they could take him home. Cheryl hoped now it would be only three or four more months.

I was amazed at Cheryl's high morale and good humor in the face of such adversity, but it was clear she was that kind of person—dogged and determined, unwilling to let anything stand in the way of what she wanted. And they wanted that baby, whom they already loved. No matter what it took, he would be theirs. I didn't know if I had the strength and stamina to go through what Cheryl and Richard had, but I assumed that a foreign adoption was the most likely route to finding an adoptable infant. I had heard that it was next to impossible to get a newborn Caucasian baby through an agency, that people spent years on agency waiting lists. As I began my investigation, I came across a newspaper article called "The Adoption Crisis" that bore this out.

According to the article, adoption agencies were overwhelmed with requests for infants—there were about a hundred hopeful adopters for every adoptable baby. Furthermore, the age cutoff for most agencies was 35; if you were over 40, forget it. The agencies did have plenty of older children and children with special needs (physical and emotional problems), but as I read about these children, I felt uncomfortable and guilty. If I wanted a child so badly, why not take one of them?

The article also mentioned private adoption, a process that usually did not involve an agency. Through private, or independent, adoption, parents of all ages were able to get newborns of any race born right here in the United States. The adoptive parents and the birth parents made the arrangements themselves, usually hiring a lawyer or lawyers to handle the legal matters. The state still had to approve the adoption through a home study by a social worker, usually after the child was already with its adoptive family. The birth mother generally gave up the baby immediately after it was born, but there was a legal period in which she could change her mind and regain custody.

I had heard about private adoption but assumed it was prohibitively expensive. The one couple I knew who had adopted this way were quite wealthy—a friend told me they had paid $25,000 to get their beautiful baby boy. The article referred to the possibility of such costs, but it said that most private adoptions ran between $5000 and $15,000 and that usually couples were able to find babies within a year or two.

I was amazed at what I read about private adoption and showed the article to Bill. I told him I was not ready for what Cheryl was going through in trying to get a baby out of a foreign country. And for the first time, I admitted to him that, although I would probably love a foreign baby, I really wanted a blonde, blue-eyed baby that looked like us. Was it really possible to find such an infant?

Seeking further information about private adoption, I called Beverly, my prefertile buddy from my exercise class. The last time I had seen her at aerobics, Beverly was bursting with excitement about a baby to be born in two weeks whom she and David would adopt. I didn't have time to get the full story, but she did tell me they would be going to Oklahoma to pick up the baby and that the whole thing had been set up by a wonderful lawyer in Tulsa. Later, she had called to tell me that they had a new baby girl, blonde, blue-eyed, and beautiful, and that they were ecstatic. We hadn't connected since then, so I called her and went over for a visit.

Lacey was 3 months old, bright-eyed, and truly gorgeous.

She already radiated her mother's vibrant energy, waving her arms, smiling, and cooing. Beverly proudly showed me the picture album they had put together of Lacey's adoption— setting up the nursery, flying to Oklahoma, picking up the baby at the hospital, and then having to stay an extra day after a tornado canceled their flight back.

I was somewhat confused about how all this had come about, so Beverly told me about the lawyer who had arranged the adoption, who, it seemed, had been handling private adoptions for about thirty years. Over the past several years, he had become "the stork" to a network of twenty or thirty families in Northern California. Beverly and David had been referred to him by a couple David knew from work who had adopted through him. What was also unusual was that this lawyer handled everything—finding the birth mother and taking care of all the legal matters—for a fee of only $1500. In total, Lacey's adoption had cost them about $12,000: They had had to pay the birth mother's prenatal and maternity medical expenses (about $500 a month of financial support for her), the fee of an adoption lawyer here in California, and travel expense to and from Oklahoma.

As I listened to Beverly and watched Lacey flapping her little arms in glee, I felt like a new world had opened up to me. I was suddenly quite nervous and wanted to ask Beverly the questions that were really on my mind: Wasn't it frightening not to know what kind of baby you'd end up with? Weren't you worried that the child might turn out to be ugly or unintelligent? But being with Beverly and Lacey, these questions seemed entirely irrelevant. Beverly was ecstatic and madly in love. "This is the most wonderful thing that has happened to me in my entire life!" she exclaimed, and I knew she meant it.

At the end of our visit, I shyly asked Beverly, "If Bill and I decide to adopt, would you refer us to the lawyer in Oklahoma?" She looked a little uncomfortable and told me I was about the tenth person to ask that. It was very difficult because he couldn't possibly find babies for everyone, and people in the network had to be very judicious with referrals. She said she'd think about it and talk to David. I left somewhat encouraged but still hoping adoption would not be necessary.

Now that we had started thinking and talking about adoption, the RESOLVE support group seemed less relevant to us. Bill and I attended only a couple more meetings, and each time we found ourselves feeling somewhat out of place. We were tired of discussing the woes of medical treatment, the insensitivity of doctors, and the anguish of failure. No one else in the group was ready to talk about adoption, which was beginning to be exciting to us.

Even though we didn't continue with the support group, RESOLVE did help us resolve our infertility. It had brought us face to face with the ghost of Christmas future. We saw ourselves becoming as tense and obsessed as these couples. We saw ourselves journeying further down the medical labyrinth, encountering ever more intense emotional and financial distress. We were ready for a new direction. We told our group leader, Camile, and she suggested we attend a RESOLVE Pre-Adoption meeting—an orientation specifically for couples interested in pursuing private adoption. A week or so later, we did.

Leading the meeting was Debra, a lawyer in her late thirties who handled private adoption cases. Her husband was also there to chime in, and a couple of times during the meeting, her towheaded daughter, about five and utterly adorable even with her thick glasses, curled up on daddy's lap to listen. She looked nothing like either of her dark-haired Jewish parents, and I wondered how they all felt about being such an incongruous family. About twenty-five of us were crammed into the living room, and we seemed to heave a quiet, collective sigh each time little Emily shuffled in and out in her footed pajamas. I saw a few tears forming when she climbed into daddy's arms to go night-night. This group was ready.

We also needed some encouragement, which Debra provided. If you were willing to put in the time and do the work, she told us, you would most likely locate a baby within a year. In fact, the average time in the private adoption cases she knew about was six to nine months. What putting in the time and doing the work meant was the ultimate in networking— sending letters out to between 1500 and 2000 people, letters that you hoped would find their way into the hands of a woman who wanted to give up her baby.

You begin by contacting everyone you know personally everywhere in the country, and then you start sending letters to anyone who might have a connection to a potential birth mother—doctors and nurses, lawyers, clergy, high school and college counselors. Some people have good results advertising in college newspapers or even in city newspapers where such ads are legal. And a number of adoption entrepreneurs sell various lists, some of them already printed on mailing labels. One list Debra knew of cost $250 for 1500 names.

Debra advised that in pursuing this process, you should work with an attorney who handles adoptions and is sensitive to all the issues involved. The attorney can serve as a go-between, and you may want to give out only his or her number on your letters. He or she also handles the legal procedures throughout the adoption period. In California, the adoption period is at least six months from the time the petition is filed, and during this period a birth mother has the right to try to reclaim the child should she change her mind. In some states, the birth father also has rights to reclaim the child, but generally he is not involved.

A private adoption can cost anywhere from $5000 to $15,000, depending on lawyers' fees, medical expenses, and living expenses for the birth mother. She is entitled legally to

"reasonable" living and medical expenses, including counseling, but some birth mothers make unreasonable demands
and get away with it; couples have been known to buy cars
and pay off back bills in order to get a baby. A scrupulous
lawyer will seek to protect you and the mother against such
abuses. All monies are paid into a trust account and distrib-
uted by the attorney. Most insurance companies will not pay
for medical expenses associated with adoptive babies, but we
were advised to check it out.

Having heard the basic overview of the private adoption
process, the group jumped right into asking questions about
lists and letters—the paper path to finding a baby. We were
given a very thorough packet of information that included
some sample letters. Apparently, the letter writing had developed into a rather precise science, since all the letters were
similar—one page long with a picture of the couple attached.
I noticed that quite a few of the pictures included the family
dog (an enticement to dog-loving teenagers?). A few had the
same opening line: "Dear birth mother, It is difficult to write
a letter to someone we have never met, and I'm sure this is a
difficult decision for you to make. We hope this letter will
make your decision a little easier."

The next paragraph described the couple's unsuccessful
attempts at conceiving a child and their intense desire to have
a family. Then there was a description of their situation: hometown, house, neighborhood, extended family, and so forth,
and some information about each hopeful parent, followed by
a paragraph about how excited they and their families were
about adopting. The final paragraph gave information about
how to reach them, usually through the lawyer or adoption
counselor—CALL COLLECT ANYTIME. Some couples were
identified just by their first name and address, some gave last
name and phone number as well.

As I looked at the letters, I marveled at the ability to
condense a life story as well as years of suffering, frustration,

and hope into five or six paragraphs. I was also struck by how all of us, reduced to these black blocks on white paper, came out sounding exactly the same. We all had faced heartbreak; we were all wonderful people with wonderful homes; we all wanted a child to love. How did a birth mother choose among Betty and Frank, Ken and Margaret, and Mary and Bill?

After we talked letters, we talked horror stories. First there is the painful process of being "interviewed" by a birth mother and being turned down—yet another painful rejection piled on top of your body's rejection of pregnancy. Then there is the awful possibility that the birth mother who chooses you will change her mind and decide to keep the baby. This may happen before the birth or at birth, in which case you have no recourse. You may end up having paid for a pregnancy and birth and still have no baby. But worse is when the birth mother changes her mind after the adoptive couple has taken possession of the child. If she has not signed the consent forms, she can reclaim her baby. In California, she has six months in which to change her mind. Every couple must be prepared for the fact that a baby they have nurtured for days, weeks, or even months can be taken away, a loss that is often emotionally devastating.

In this room full of emotional survivors, that terrible eventuality seemed a small risk. As we shared our thoughts about adoption, almost everyone was ready to go ahead with the paper chase. Some couples already had their letters out, and at the breaks we questioned each other about lists and locations most likely to produce results.

Bill and I left excited but somewhat stunned by what lay ahead of us. I was now in my busiest monsoon season of work, as was Bill. The thought of taking on the letter-writing project overwhelmed us. The other major concern was our house. We had bought a very small house in a lovely location planning to remodel it, and we had only one bedroom (two small rooms downstairs could be reached only by going outside). We were planning to start the addition that spring. If we did get a baby, he or she would have to be in our bedroom and then live through months of construction. Maybe this wasn't the time. Maybe we should wait until the house was all done, until Bill's business was making more money, until we could be sure we weren't going to get pregnant ourselves.

Over the next week or so, waves of doubt and desire washed over each of us. We knew we wanted a child, but were we ready for adoption? If we did get the letters out soon, it might be a year, but then again it could be a few months or a few weeks. We still had more intrauterine inseminations to do—what if I got pregnant during the adoption process? What about the costs? We had just refinanced our house and were able to get out $10,000 in cash. That might cover adoption costs, but it could also pay for more fertility treatment—for two in vitro fertilizations if we decided to go that route. If we did adopt, how would our families react—would they feel completely comfortable with a baby we did not bear?

We also discussed the issue of "open adoption" raised in the RESOLVE meeting. We understood that in an open adoption, the birth mother generally chose the adoptive couple and both parties met each other at some point. They might get to know each other only slightly, or they might maintain contact throughout the pregnancy. The adoptive couple who ran the meeting knew their birth mother well and were thrilled, in fact, that she had just called them about adopting a second baby she was pregnant with. She had lived with them during the last months of her pregnancy, and they had been present at the birth. They believed that open adoption was best for all parties as long as the birth parents and the adoptive parents agreed on the kind of relationship they wanted to have. In some open adoptions, the birth mother became a central figure in her child's life. In others, pictures and phone calls were exchanged once or twice a year.

The important thing in open adoption was that all parties

in the adoption triad knew each other. The adoptive child knew who his or her biological parents were and why they gave him or her up and therefore would not suffer from adoption identity problems. The birth parents were able to resolve their grief and guilt by knowing their child and his or her life circumstances. The adoptive parents would not have to face future problems with children being obsessed about or searching for their "real parents."

The picture our group leaders painted of open adoption sounded good, but where did you draw the line in the relationship? We had no place in our home for a pregnant woman, and we wanted to adopt an infant, not an infant and a teenager. What might open adoption get us into? We tried to think about adoption from a birth mother's point of view—acknowledging the pain, uncertainty, and guilt that must surround giving up a baby just born to you. Would it truly be easier if she knew she could maintain some contact with her child or know personally the people who would be its mother and father? Or would it only aggravate an already difficult situation, denying or postponing what must inevitably be a process of letting go? Wouldn't the birth mother be more likely to try to get her baby back if she spent time with him or her? Might not the whole situation turn into one big entanglement? We admitted to each other that we'd prefer not to have an ongoing personal relationship with the birth parents but that we did feel it would be good to communicate with them yearly with letters and pictures if that's what they wanted. Still, the open adoption situation seemed far away.

Our questions about adoption continued to ebb and flow, until one evening we received a phone call from Jordan, Bill's oldest and best friend on the East Coast. We had visited him and his wife, Gloria, a few months earlier in Washington, D.C. At that time, Gloria had recently found out she was pregnant, and we celebrated over Cuban food in one of the city's myriad ethnic restaurants. But now the cause for celebration was over.

Jordan told us in a hushed voice that their baby was dead. Gloria had had some problems with the pregnancy and had been hospitalized. When she went into labor prematurely, a sonogram revealed that the baby's lungs had not developed. In the process of birth, the baby died. There had been no way to save him.

Who ever knows what to say? We could only tell them how sorry we were, that we knew how devastated they were, and that we would be thinking of them. But as we thought of Jordan and Gloria, their baby and their grief, what we began to feel was our own devastation and sadness. That night, as Bill and I held each other and cried, we realized for the first time that we too were mourning the death of a child—the child we were not able to bring to life. How could we mourn what we had never had? He or she had been alive in our fantasies and dreams for two years; he or she had been the focus of our lives. We grieved not for what had been, but for what would not be.

For several days, the grief stayed with me, shrouding my heart and putting me back in touch with my father's death thirty-four years ago when I was 7. I remembered lying in bed the night he died, staring at the ceiling and saying over and over to myself, "It isn't true. . . . this didn't happen. . . . I'll wake up in the morning and he'll be there." I didn't go to my father's funeral. My mother and grandparents thought I was too young, and I certainly didn't insist on going. I didn't want to believe he was really dead. In a way, I didn't really accept his death until I was in my twenties, going through psychotherapy. Finally, all the anger and grief emerged and was expressed, and I began to feel whole for the first time in my life.

Gradually, I realized that the process of our infertility was similar to the emotional experience of death. During the past two years, I had experienced denial, anger, guilt, depression, and grief—all the stages one goes through in confronting death. I had pretended there was no problem—"Next month

I'll get pregnant." I had been angry at myself, at the doctors, at Bill, at God, and at my fertile friends. I had blamed myself for not "creating the reality" of having a child. And God knows, I'd been depressed, feeling listless about my life and the future. During all these stages, I had cried, but I had not truly grieved. Just as I had kept my father with me all those years, I had refused to let go of my unborn child.

Yes, it is hard to grieve for something that never existed. There is no funeral and no grave. There are no flowers, no friends offering comfort and support. There is, literally, nothing to cry about. There is only an abstract loss, but it is a loss nonetheless—the loss of a dream. For a few days, I mourned our loss. Bill, too, felt the sadness of letting go of our natural child. He acknowledged for the first time his sense of failure, that he had not been able to give me what I wanted most in the world. He had not been able to "make everything all right." That week we felt very close to each other, very tentative and vulnerable, but soon our strength returned. Grieving for our unborn child became a turning point in our decision about adoption. Our tears seemed to have washed away our confusion and fear, and we felt ready to move on.

I called Beverly and asked if Bill and I could come for a visit. I wanted Bill to meet her, David, and Lacey, and for us all to talk about adoption. I also wanted to find out more about their adoption lawyer in Oklahoma. Perhaps if they got to know us better, they would consider referring us to him.

That hope made us a little nervous about the visit—our first audition to become adoptive parents. In true Yuppie tradition, we brought a quiche to brunch at their house, a beautiful brown-shingle overlooking Mt. Tamalpais. We cooed over Lacey until she took her morning nap and then had a long conversation with Beverly and David about adoption. We voiced our concerns about timing, about our small house, and about our feelings of financial insecurity. Bill talked about wanting a foreign baby; I said I wanted one just like Lacey. We expressed our reservations about open adoption, which they shared. They had had no contact with Lacey's birth mother and were grateful she had not wanted any involvement with them. To all of our concerns they responded warmly and openly, in essence telling us that the time would never be right to have a baby, that you just had to take the leap. They had shared all our' fears about adoption, and now those fears seemed far in the past. Lacey fulfilled every dream they had of a child and more. "Don't wait," David urged us. "Just go for it!"

They talked cautiously about their lawyer during our visit, but they also gave us information about other private adoption sources. They showed us the letter they had prepared but never sent out. We didn't quite understand the lawyer's role —was he certain to find a baby for you? Yes, he would find babies for couples referred to him, but how long it would take would depend on his waiting list. They had been prepared to send out letters as well but had decided just to wait for word from Oklahoma. It was only a matter of months from the time they were referred to him until he called about Lacey's birth mother.

I couldn't believe it could be that easy. At the end of our visit, I got up the nerve to ask straight out, "Would you both consider referring us to your lawyer in Oklahoma?" There was a long pause as they looked at each other. They would talk it over, they said, and let us know soon.

A few days later, Beverly called to say she had contacted their lawyer, Scott Roberts, about us and that he was expecting to hear from us regarding adoption. He had a few people ahead of us on his list, and he had no idea when it might happen. The prospects came irregularly—sometimes one or two in a month, sometimes none for several months. Probably, he would find a baby for us within the next nine months.

Chapter Five

❦

Adopting Alexander

*T*he idea that Scott Roberts of Tulsa, Oklahoma,* was going to find a baby for us within the next nine months seemed too good to be true. Was this really happening? Could we trust it? Was nine months an average time? Could it take longer? Maybe we should start sending out our own letters just in case—at least to friends and family throughout the country. We had to send Scott a picture and letter that would go to potential birth mothers, so we decided to make it appropriate for a mass mailing should one be necessary. I worked on the letter for a week, revising it again and again with Bill's help and some input from Beverly. It read:

> We are a happy, loving couple seeking to adopt an
> infant to love and raise as our own. We have been

---

*Not his real name or location.

91

trying to get pregnant for over two years, but extensive fertility treatment has yielded no diagnosis and no results. It has been a very frustrating experience; but now, having decided to adopt, we are thrilled with the prospect of at last having the family we have dreamed of.

Bill and I met three years ago, fell in love (at first sight), and married in June, 1984. Our love continues to grow and deepen, and we feel we have a perfect partnership for creating a happy, loving, and stable environment for children.

A little about ourselves: We are both college-educated and come from close, loving families. Bill was born and raised in the Midwest. After several years as a psychotherapist, he became a builder and is now a general contractor and owner of a small construction company. The company is growing rapidly because of the quality of his work and his wonderful way with people. Bill also has a delightfully playful way with kids and is looking forward to sharing his energy and creativity with our children.

I, Mary, was born and raised in the South and was also a psychotherapist and high school teacher. For the past eight years I have been a free-lance writer and media producer, working on film, video, and multi-image productions. Although my work is creative and challenging, I am now most excited about devoting myself to being a mother. I plan to be at home with the baby, with work as a secondary focus.

Bill and I live in a lovely home nestled among the trees in a small town just north of San Francisco. Ours is a tightly-knit neighborhood, ideal for raising kids. We are very fortunate to be co-owners (with three other families) of a large swimming pool and to have a beautiful garden of vegetables and flowers. Within walking distance of our home are woods, hiking trails, a public park, tennis courts, and an elementary school that is considered one of the best in the country.

We lead an active life outdoors (swimming, tennis, scuba-diving, hiking, gardening, and skiing) and indoors (reading, movies, cooking). We look forward to sharing these interests as well as our love for music and travel with our children. We are blessed with wonderful friends and a close extended family, all of whom are enthusiastic about the prospect of our adopting a baby.

Bill and I have an extraordinarily strong relationship based on deep love and affection. More than anything, we want to share our love with a child and create an environment in which our child can achieve his or her natural potential.

We hope you know of a child for us. We have a great deal to give. Please call us collect anytime at home (number) or, if you prefer, contact our adoption lawyer, Scott Roberts, (number).

Along with the letter, I sent a picture of us taken the night before our wedding. Bill was in a suit and I was in a strapless white dress. I was worried that we looked too dressed up and formal—not "homey" enough, but it was a great picture of us, glowing with a love we hoped would be apparent to a young woman with child. Meanwhile, we joked about who our birth parents might be and had various silly fantasies, such as a mother who was an ex-Miss Oklahoma studying nuclear physics and a father who was a star University of Oklahoma quarterback with a Rhodes Scholarship.

The fantasy reflected my misgivings about adoption, however. Whose gene pool would we be dipping into? I still couldn't imagine that our adopted baby could be as great as a little MaryBill, but I tried not to think about it. I was glad we would have several months to get used to the idea and also to continue with fertility treatment. We had another IUI coming up, and maybe it would work. Even though I felt I had gone through one level of grieving the loss of our biological child, I still hoped that he or she would yet appear. I thought of the "Give it up and then it comes to you" syndrome. Clearly, I had not totally given up. I prayed insemination number four would be the lucky one.

A few days after the insemination, and about a week after we sent the letter and picture to Scott Roberts, Beverly called me at work. I was in the midst of a big production push, finishing up a multi-image show to take to Washington the next day. "Get ready for this," she said. Scott had just called her about a potential baby. I guess he wanted her to call to feel us out, since he didn't know us yet and didn't know how we'd feel about the situation. A young woman had come to him who was pregnant by a Vietnamese man. The baby was not due for six or seven months, but she was sure she wanted to give it up for adoption. Were we interested?

I didn't know what to say. My mind was crying no! I'm not ready yet! I don't really want to have to adopt! I want to get pregnant! But I couldn't say it out loud. I just stammered about how this was really fast and I'd have to talk to Bill. I think Beverly sensed my reaction and told me we should know that we had absolutely no obligation to take this particular baby. Scott had emphasized that fact to her. She knew Bill was interested in an Asian child, so she wanted us to know about it. Talk to Bill, she said, and then call Scott directly.

I was flushed with anxiety when I called Bill. He, too, was surprised at something happening so quickly and suggested I call Scott directly to get more information. Scott answered the phone with an Okie drawl and began talking nonstop. He was happy to have us as clients, he said, and he had put us near the top of his list because of my age. Then he told me what he knew about the birth mother and her situation but kept saying it was fine if we decided not to go with this opportunity. I almost felt he was intimating that this wasn't right for us, but he was scrupulous in giving us all the information he had and letting us decide. I told him we'd call him the next day.

Driving back home across the Golden Gate Bridge, I thought and I cried. Why wasn't I thrilled about this half-Vietnamese baby? Here was probably the fastest, easiest adoption in the world staring me in the face and I was balking. Did I really not want a child? Despite all my ideals, was I really a racist at heart? Bill would probably think this was great, and we'd end up divided. Could I really love a child who looked nothing like me? If we passed on this baby, how long would we have to wait for another? Think how many couples would be overjoyed with this opportunity! How could we say no? But how could we say yes? Even though I didn't feel anything, I could be pregnant this very minute. Before Bill got home, I sat on the bed and meditated, asking God or my Higher Self to tell us what to do.

I was surprised to hear a voice in my head clearly say, "This is not your child." I didn't trust it, feeling it must be my fear talking. But the voice seemed calm and certain. When Bill got home and we finally sat down and looked into each other's eyes, I was surprised to see that he was as scared as I was. This wasn't his idea of a foreign child, he said. If we were going to get a baby of another race, he wanted one who was actually from another part of the world. And besides, this was just too fast; he wasn't ready either. He held me close and I told him about my meditation. We agreed to call Scott and tell him that we'd pass on this baby. The next day, Scott told us he thought we'd made the right decision and that he was sure there would be another baby soon.

The flurry of travel, running the multi-image show in Washington, and a brief trip home to North Carolina gave us little time to think about our decision. But on the flight back home, we started questioning it. Had we acted out of fear? Were we stupid not to take this baby? During a layover, we put in a call to Scott but couldn't reach him. The next day, Beverly called to tell us that one of the women in the California network had friends who had just been through their third miscarriage and had decided to adopt. The woman was Japanese and the man Caucasian. Coincidentally, their friend had called Scott about them the very day we passed on the baby. Scott had contacted them immediately, and they were unbelievably thrilled with the prospect of getting a newborn Asian-Caucasian baby—almost unheard of in the adoption world. When I heard the news, something inside me shifted. It seemed that this match was perfect and that my inner voice had spoken the truth.

Even though I felt we'd made the right decision about the baby we passed on, the incident left us feeling unsettled about adoption and whether we were really ready. It had added a dimension of seriousness to our lives (this business of adopting a child is for keeps!) and also revealed the depth of our insecurities. I talked at length to my mother, who was disappointed we hadn't taken the baby but was certain that the right baby would come to us soon and that we'd better get ourselves ready. My mother, a long-time believer in metaphysics, had often told me that we "choose" our parents and our children—that there are mystical forces at work that bring together the beings who belong together. I began to wonder about a soul out there destined to come to Mary and Bill Chase, a being who was waiting for a passionate teenage liaison somewhere in Oklahoma to give it an opportunity to come to life.

The desire to believe that fate was at work and that "our baby" would find us led me again to the world of metaphysics. I wanted some advice, and a friend of mine suggested I try to talk to Lazaris. If you know about Shirley MacLaine's spiritual exploits, you'll understand about Lazaris. He is a being without a body who is channeled through a trance medium. Jach, a real person, goes into a trance and speaks as Lazaris, who represents another level of human consciousness. Lazaris is a well-known and well-respected entity in the world of channelers and had been working with people primarily in the San Francisco Bay Area for more than ten years. Over the years, I had attended several Lazaris workshops and gatherings. I wasn't sure what I believed about Lazaris and who was talking, a disembodied entity or Jach, the channel. Whatever or whoever was talking, I always found the messages and teachings powerful, relevant, and enjoyable. Lazaris has a great sense of humor and deep insight into the human psyche.

It was almost impossible to get an appointment to talk to Lazaris, as he was booked years in advance, but I knew my friend Helen had regular appointments with him. I asked her if she would be willing to take a few minutes to speak to Lazaris about our baby situation. Specifically, I wanted her to ask him what was in the way of our getting pregnant and whether we should adopt. If we did adopt, what should we be aware of? She said she'd try to fit our questions into their next session.

The message that came back from Lazaris was both disturbing and encouraging. Bill and I listened anxiously to Helen's tape of the session. Lazaris said that nothing was physically wrong with either of us but that there was a lot of tension around getting pregnant—unconscious fears associated with my age. He mentioned the dangers of pregnancy and the possibility of Down's syndrome. Oh no, I thought, is this going to be another one of those "just relax and it will happen" lectures? He suggested examining those fears but moved quickly to talking about adoption. Yes, he felt very positive about the adoption, but first we had to clear away our feelings of failure. We had to recognize that the soul of the person meant to be our child would get to us no matter whose body it came through, mine or someone else's. We should consciously "program" our reality. That meant we should meditate on adopting with two affirmations: "The consciousness that wants to be ours will come to us," and "The parents of our child will be healthy." He also said that we should pick and choose, that we should not feel we have to take any baby that came along, but rather we should pay attention to what felt right to us. If we approached the adoption consciously, he said, the "right" baby would come. Furthermore, that baby would look like us no matter what his biological parents looked like. "Children look like their parents not just because of genes," he said, "but because they want to." He ended by saying that if we did decide to adopt, we might find ourselves pregnant in the future. "Be sure to use birth control if you don't want a second child."

What to make of all this? I felt annoyed at the suggestion that my infertility was "all in my mind," and I was not aware of any overwhelming fears about problems with pregnancy or birth—I didn't feel any more afraid than anyone else would. But what Lazaris said about our adoption was very encouraging, and I hoped it was true. I liked the idea of "creating" our adoption as we wanted it to be, bringing in the soul destined to be ours. Perhaps my mother was right—that we do choose each other. We sort of scoffed at the notion of a child's looking like us because it wanted to, but who knew? We also liked the idea of getting pregnant after adopting. (Wasn't that what everyone said happens?) Although the conversation with Lazaris hadn't really given us any specific answers, it moved us further toward feeling positive about adopting—an inner sense that maybe this whole thing would work out after all.

We moved from being positive to being downright excited after we attended the annual reunion of families in the Scott Roberts adoption network. It was about a month after we had made it to "the list," and Marie, the woman who had started the network, kindly invited us to join the party and meet Scott and his wife in person. We drove an hour to Fremont, on the other side of the bay, and entered a house literally brimming with children—babes in arms, toddlers, and kids up to age 10 crawled, ran, jumped, squealed, and hollered among about thirty to forty adoptive parents.

When we first walked in the door and were welcomed with champagne, we saw a huge poster of pictures entitled "SCOTT ROBERTS FAMILY TREE." Marie, her husband, Carl, and their four kids, three of whom were adopted, were at the top. Underneath the pictures of their kids, the tree branched off to pictures of kids adopted by families they had referred to Scott. The branching continued through several generations, and at the bottom, connected by lines to their referring friends, was a list of couples entitled "EXPECTING." Second on the list were "Bill and Mary Chase." Bill and I looked at our names and then at each other. My husband's eyes were filled with tears.

A few minutes later, we met Scott in person, a gregarious blond man in his fifties who was working the crowd like a master politician, kissing babies, hugging women, and telling off-color jokes to the men. We weren't quite prepared for such an outrageous personality, but we liked him immediately, and it seemed he liked us. There wasn't much chance to talk, as everyone was grabbing him for hugs and conversation, so we just watched, marveling at this man who would be our "stork." We met Margaret, Mrs. Stork, who was immobilized with a broken foot—a warm, beautiful woman who made us feel wonderfully welcomed into "the family." The only people we knew there were Beverly and David and little Lacey, but everyone made us feel very comfortable.

The next few hours were mindboggling. We met a dozen or more adoptive parents with children of all ages. It was uncanny how much these children resembled their parents: No one would have guessed these families were all biologically unrelated. I had thought that Lazaris's statement about adopted children choosing to look like their parents was silly, but now I began to wonder.... Also present and listed as "expecting" were George and Doris, the couple who would be adopting the half-Vietnamese baby we had passed on. I wasn't sure if they knew about our involvement with their child-to-be, so we didn't mention it and just talked about how excited they must be to be "due" in five months.

After a potluck feast, we gathered in the living room, and Scott became master of ceremonies for "awards" he made to various folks, including our hosts and Philip Adams,* his legal counterpart in California. Like Scott, Philip was a full-fledged character. Well into his eighties, he had a full head of hair, an oversized plaid bow tie, and an attractive wife half his age. Phil Adams, we learned, had been doing adoptions in California for over forty years and had a lot to do with the state's adoption laws. In his awards ceremony, Scott made Phil an honorary Okie—complete with a certificate signed by the governor and a very fine cowboy hat, a neat complement to the huge plaid bow tie. To each of the families present he gave a calligraphed poem, "Legacy of an Adopted Child," which ends with this verse:

> *And now you ask me through your tears,*
> *the age-old questions through the years;*
> *Heredity or environment—which are you the product*
> *   of?*
> *Neither, my darling, neither—just two different kinds*
> *   of love.*

Eyes welled with tears and noses sniffled as Scott read the poem out loud. We felt the love that made this reunion such an extraordinary event and could hardly believe we were so lucky as to be a part of it. Were there other networks like

---

*His real name.

this? It just seemed so incredible that one person had brought so much happiness to all these families! Driving home, we were both glowing with the warmth of a newfound family, and we kept looking at each other and saying "we're expecting!"

A few days later, I had insemination number five, and though my hopes were not high, I found myself wishing we would become just a great story to the Oklahoma adoption network—the couple who got pregnant right after being referred to Scott. Within a week, I knew I was not pregnant, but it was not as hard to take now. We would have a family. It was only a matter of time. We started collecting books of baby names and poring over them at bedtime. We both agreed we wanted a girl and that we would name her Alexandra. We also like Alexander for a boy.

During Thanksgiving and Christmas, we began to feel comfortable enough to tell friends "we're expecting." At a big holiday banquet and dance, we found ourselves seated next to a young woman, Beth, whom I'd known years before. When we told her about our plans to adopt, she told us that several years ago when she was single and unemployed, she had given up a baby for adoption. I braced for a sob story about how painful it had been for her but was surprised when she told us it had been a wonderful experience. She had heard about private adoption, contacted Phil Adams, and ended up choosing a couple who were clients of his. She met them prior to the birth but told them she did not want any contact with her child—that they were the "real" parents and should refer to her as "the birth lady." She said she felt the term "birth mother" was misleading and might confuse the child with the idea of having two mothers. For her, giving a childless couple her baby was a joyous contribution, and she continued to feel good about her decision. She knew she had done the right thing for her child. We were moved by Beth's happy account of the other side of the adoption scene. We hoped so much that the mother of our child-to-be would feel as Beth had and that our joy in receiving a child would not mean pain for the woman giving it up.

During this time, we also gave ourselves a break from fertility treatment for a couple of months. Although I still made sure we made love right around ovulation, we actually got to have sex with each other rather than with white cups and tubes. What a relief! I began to remember what great sex could be like—spontaneous and anxiety-free. Other aspects of life seemed to benefit from our renewed energy as well. We were both working a lot, saving some money, and beginning to meet with an architect about expanding our house.

We also had a new adventure to distract us. Someone at *Life* magazine had seen my article about "Waiting for Baby" in the *San Francisco Chronicle*. Ruth, a *Life* reporter, had called a couple of months earlier to ask if she could feature us in an issue of the magazine devoted to infertility and what couples will go through to have children. She was particularly interested in the "unusual" steps we'd taken, such as seeing an acupuncturist, drinking herbs, talking to psychics, rebirthing, and meditating.

Although Ruth seemed to be a genuine and sensitive person, I could tell right away that *Life* was likely to feature us as the "California kooks" who would do anything, no matter how stupid, to have a baby. I made sure Ruth understood that the focus of our fertility treatment had been medical rather than metaphysical and that any story about us would have to make that clear. Bill and I talked over the possibility of our story being trivialized or made fun of, but we decided we'd accept the invitation. Neither of us had to worry about any consequences from looking silly. If the article gave anyone anywhere permission to be more open with themselves and others about their infertility and to try nonmedical approaches, then it would be worth it. And, of course, our egos weren't immune to a little publicity. We liked the idea of being photographed for a national magazine and hoped it would be fun.

On February 1, a few days before the *Life* team was scheduled to arrive for a three-day shoot, we got a message on our machine to call Scott Roberts. We knew it must be news of a baby. We had just driven back from Los Angeles and it was after midnight, so we had to wait until the next day to call. Bill hugged me and seemed genuinely happy. I could hardly sleep, uncertain whether I was feeling excitement or fear.

When we called Scott, he matter-of-factly drawled the story of a young girl who'd come to see him with her mother last week. Eileen was 18, a senior in high school in a Tulsa suburb, and about six months pregnant. Supposedly, she had conceived the night she lost her virginity—at a party the summer before. She had been raised as a Catholic and evidently hadn't considered abortion, but she had kept her pregnancy a secret for nearly six months. Wearing baggy clothes worked for a while, but she finally told her mother. Now they both agreed that it was best to give the baby up for adoption. Scott described Eileen as 5 feet, 3 inches, about 120 pounds, with dark brown hair and dark eyes—"about a seven on a scale of ten" (his usual rating scale of general attractiveness).

According to Scott, Eileen came from a "good family." Both parents were professionals but had been divorced for some time. She seemed to be an intelligent, responsible girl who didn't drink, smoke, or take drugs. Her medical history revealed she was in good health, and there were no health problems in the family. He was concerned that she hadn't had any prenatal care, but a doctor's exam indicated all was going well with the pregnancy. She would be having a sonogram the next day, and we might know whether the baby was a boy or a girl.

Most important, Eileen seemed very certain about giving

up the baby. She had a friend who had gotten pregnant and kept the baby, and she'd witnessed what a burden it was. Scott described her as sort of a happy-go-lucky girl, who laughed and joked with him some and didn't seem too upset about her condition. She would continue with school so she could graduate and would be living at home, so we wouldn't have to pay for living expenses. The only problem for us might be that she would not identify the baby's father. All she would say was that he was Caucasian, about 21, and 6 feet tall with light brown hair. She said she hadn't seen him since that fateful night and didn't want to involve him at all. Scott had not pushed her to identify him, since it would have meant having to get the father's permission, which could cause bigger problems. Unless we felt we had to know about him, he would let it be.

Scott, as we knew from Beverly and David, was not a fan of open adoption. He believed that all parties were better off without any contact with one another—that contact only led to complications. He had told Eileen and her mother about us and had answered their questions. We didn't know whether she knew anything about open adoption, but Scott reported that she didn't want to meet us. He said she preferred that the baby go out of state, so she wouldn't have to worry about running into her child. "This looks like a real good situation," he said, and, gasping, we agreed.

The story rushed over us like a tidal wave, and when we hung up we were both shaking—Bill with excitement and me with fear. He was jubilant, and although I wanted to share his enthusiasm, I found myself feeling completely terrified. This was the real thing—an undeniably wonderful adoption opportunity due the end of April. Why was I so sad and scared? I tried to act happy, but Bill knew I was not. He didn't try to change me or push me, knowing how I react to pressure. Lovingly, he just let me be.

I had thought that I was completely ready for a baby to

come to us, but now I was terrified. I spent the next few days afraid and disoriented, trying to face up to my deeply uncomfortable resistance. First I had to admit to myself how disappointed I was that Eileen had brown eyes and hair and that she was not a "ten." I knew the Miss Oklahoma fantasy was a joke, but I found I was very attached to the idea of having a baby that would look like us. I was embarrassed to tell anyone I felt that way except Bill and my mother. When I called Mother to tell her about Eileen, she was thrilled. I was unnerved. I suppose I wanted her to support my doubts, but instead she was completely enthusiastic. "But Mother," I whined, "the baby won't look like us. She (I was still counting on a girl) will have brown eyes and brown hair." Her response: "Well, you know how to make her hair blonde—you've been doing it to yourself for twenty years!"

The next jolt came a couple of days later when Scott called to tell us that the sonogram had revealed the baby was a boy. I should have been thrilled that he was reported to be in great shape, but instead I was disappointed. No bows in the hair and sweet little dresses, just jeans and T-shirts. The house would be littered with trucks and transformers instead of dolls and tea sets. Oh, well, at least we wouldn't have to buy Barbie doll outfits.

I kept questioning Scott about Eileen: Was she smart in school? What grades did she get? Was she nice-looking? Was her hair curly or straight? Scott said he would send a picture of her, but I was afraid to see it. What if I didn't like her looks? I was so ashamed of my petty feelings, I didn't talk about them with Scott. I knew that there were thousands and thousands of couples who would be overjoyed to be in the position of receiving a newborn baby with such ease. What was going on with me? How could I get past this fear?

I began by calling Beverly and confessing my ambivalence. She was understanding and empathetic, telling me she'd been terrified, too. It's a powerful shock, she said, to

confront your own narcissism and the "pictures" you hang on
to that define who you are. She acknowledged how difficult
it was to really let go of having your own genetic child. I told
her we felt we had already grieved the loss of our biological
child, but she reminded me that grieving is often like peeling
an onion: You may find you have layer after layer of sadness.
She also reminded me that if we didn't feel ready, we didn't
have to take this baby—that we were not riding some irre-
versible current. We had every right to take more time if we
needed to.

I called three other women who had adopted, one of
whom I had not met but who was a friend of a friend. They
all knew what I was going through and acknowledged their
own fears and petty concerns (though they hardly seemed as
petty as mine). They had worried primarily about the baby's
health and intelligence and, of course, about whether the
mother would change her mind. That fear had not struck me
yet, but I figured I would probably get around to it. A couple
of women, like Beverly, said they had felt totally unprepared
for motherhood and worried about their ability to care for a
baby. When she first got her baby, Marianne freaked out over
the scab around the navel where the cord had been cut. She
thought it was a disease and called the hospital emergency
room in the middle of the night. Penny, frantically trying to
prepare for her baby's arrival, had found herself wandering
through Macy's baby department crying because she didn't
know what to buy. Finally, she just stood in the aisle and
started yelling "Help!" and a nice grandma came to her aid.

All the adoptive mothers also told me the same thing:
Once the baby is in your arms, no matter who or what it looks
like, it will be yours. You will fall in love immediately, and
there will never be a doubt about its being your baby. Jane,
who had found her adopted baby through a newspaper ad in
Oregon, was particularly understanding and encouraging. She
and her husband are both blonde and blue-eyed, while their

daughter Victoria has black eyes and hair. They fell madly in love with Victoria the minute they saw her and couldn't imagine loving her any more than they did. For Jane and the other two adoptive mothers, the bonding process happened almost instantaneously, with no doubts or questions or regrets. I heard what these women had to say and felt better, but I still could not shake my fear and an underlying sense of sadness.

Bill continued to be positive about the baby, but since he could tell my enthusiasm was being choked off by something, he remained fairly subdued. He could hardly believe that it was true—that something this monumental was coming about so easily. He was not concerned whether the baby was a boy or a girl, only that it was healthy, and Eileen's clean bill of health was all he needed. But it was clear I needed to work something out, and Bill continued to let me be, giving me room to discover what fear had hold of my heart.

In the midst of all this, the *Life* magazine team arrived, and we had four days filled with photography sessions, interviews, and great dinners out courtesy of the magazine. By the end of the first day of shooting, I was certain we would be the California Kooks. My friend Evan, the Rebirther, just happened to call that day. He had just returned from visiting various South American "power spots"—just in time to reenact my rebirthing session for the cameras. At dinner he wowed the *Life* team with stories of spaceships landing and extraterrestrials among us. But we're not California kooks, we kept reminding them!

When they wanted to get shots of me getting acupunctured and drinking herbs and both of us meditating together by the Bay, we became concerned about the direction of the article and insisted that *Life* give equal time to what was really the focus of our fertility treatment—our work with Dr. B.

He was willing to come in to the office on a Saturday morning for a photo opportunity. During the setup time for various shots, Ruth interviewed him for the article and I took the opportunity to find out as much as I could about Pergonal, thinking I would take it during my next cycle. I still had one more opportunity to get pregnant before Eileen's baby was due, and I wanted to go for it. Dr. B was not very encouraging. Since it looked like I was ovulating and my tubes were clear, the Pergonal was not really a "treatment" per se, only the next available weapon in the arsenal. It might beef up my ovulation, but Dr. B thought my chances of getting pregnant on it were around 15 percent. He would certainly go ahead with it, but we shouldn't get our hopes up.

Within those first two days, the *Life* folks, Ruth and the photographer and his assistant, became intimately involved in our life, and we began to feel like friends. They knew an adoption was imminent, and I shared with them some of my fear and ambivalence. They also heard me talk about it with a psychic—an appointment arranged for the benefit of the cameras. I wasn't able to locate Angela, the psychic we'd talked to the year before, so we went to see someone who was recommended by a friend. He was a young man who was a "channel" for another-worldly being like Lazaris. It was strange enough to be talking to a being without a body in a small Berkeley apartment, but lights, cameras, photographers, and a reporter made it truly bizarre. Nevertheless, the psychic, whose alter ego called himself "Amman," gave us a very interesting perspective on our infertility. Like Lazaris, he said the problem was located "above the neck," and he attributed it to imbalances in our male and female energies. I could tell that Bill was insulted. It also didn't ring true to me, and I pursued the issue of our adoption. "Who is this being in Eileen's belly in Oklahoma, and should we go through with the adoption?" Amman told us we had known this being for many lifetimes and that we were all "good buddies." In answer to my question about how to deal with my fear and ambivalence, he gave me a regimen of meditation for the next two weeks that would enable me to come to a decision.

I managed to forget the whole thing during our last day of shooting—some shots of us running on the beach, then a trip to the bed and breakfast inn in the wine country where we'd gotten married. We were illustrating the "romantic get-away" as a surefire way to get pregnant. It was there that we took a picture of me standing on my head (supposedly right after intercourse), in the process of which I kicked Bill in the face and gave him a black eye. At least I waited until the last shot.

When the *Life* team departed, I was left again with my fear and indecision, and I knew I couldn't take two weeks out to meditate on it, as Amman had suggested. In fact, I couldn't stand it any longer. I called my friend Paula, a Reichian therapist, and asked if she would do a therapy session with me. When I had been a therapist a decade ago, I had worked primarily with the Reichian method—moving clients quickly into an emotional state by using breathing techniques similar to Rebirthing. I was ready now to stop thinking and talking about what was going on with me and go directly to the heart of the matter.

I came to Paula's office on a sunny afternoon. My heart leaned heavily on my knotted stomach, and I felt slightly sick. Paula knew what I was going through and didn't say much to me. She had me lie down on a large mattress and instructed me to begin breathing. Almost immediately, I began crying, then sobbing, then screaming. "It's not fair! God damn it, it's not fair!" Paula told me to let go and just move any way I wanted to. I clenched my fists and began to hit the mattress. I yelled and pounded until I was exhausted, and then I lay quietly for a while feeling empty. Then an image appeared in my mind of a small girl with white blonde hair. She was crying. As I looked into her blue eyes, I saw myself.

I realized then it wasn't just a child I wanted, it was a little me. I wanted to recreate a little Mary so I could change my own childhood. I wanted to give her a perfect father who wouldn't die and leave her. I wanted to give her a mother who was always happy and who would understand her completely. Through this child, I could transform my own childhood and therefore my life. Through her, I could take away the pain, the hurt, and the insecurity and make everything all right.

With insight and sensitivity, Paula helped me contact that little girl and begin to give her the love and comfort she needed. As I communicated with the child in me, I saw that only I could heal her sorrow. The healing would have to take place within myself rather than through someone else. I could not expect my child to transform my life for me. I could not expect him to bear the burden of my life as well as his own. Once I confronted this truth, I realized how wrong it would be to bring a child into the world to be another me. If there were indeed some metaphysical reason I had not gotten pregnant, perhaps it was just this lesson, that a child is his or her own person and not an extension of me.

These insights came to me quietly and tearfully as I lay on the mattress and talked with Paula. At the end of our session, my chest felt like an open window with soft breezes blowing through. The afternoon sun sparkled with new brilliance, and I knew something had shifted in me. By the time I got home, I found I was incredibly excited about our baby, our Alexander. He was no longer Eileen's baby to me. He was our child, the one we had chosen, the one who had chosen us.

I couldn't wait to tell Bill about my realizations and about how excited I now felt about Alexander. As I shared my experience encountering the child in me, Bill, too, began to cry. He was finally able to tell me how he had been feeling the past two weeks, how difficult it had been for him to contain his excitement and to try not to "snow" me with it. From the moment Scott called, he had "known" that this was our baby. He told me that he had trusted I would find the source of my misgivings, and so he had been holding back on purpose, waiting for me to come around. He didn't know what he would have done if I had not been able to get through my fears— perhaps the power of his "inner voice" and his conviction could have convinced me—but he was grateful that I had found my own path to accepting our child. We hugged and kissed and then started jumping up and down laughing and crying, "We're going to have a baby!"

The adoption started to feel very real after our first meeting with Philip Adams, who would handle the adoption process in California. Decked out in yet another great bow tie, Phil greeted us with mock gruffness: "I don't know why anyone would want a screaming baby around, but we'll go ahead with this." He explained that although our baby would come from Oklahoma, the California adoption procedures would still apply. After the baby was born, he would file a petition to adopt, and within 180 days a social worker from the State Department of Social Services would come to do a "home study," which would determine our basic fitness as parents. If the baby were born in California, the social worker would also meet with the birth mother (and birth father, if available) to discuss her decision and make sure she knew her rights. Since the consent to adoption papers would already have been signed before we left Oklahoma with the baby and we would already be his legal guardians, we shouldn't expect any problems with the final adoption. Still, it would not be final until at least six months after the petition was filed. We were relieved to hear that once the consent to adoption was signed, there was almost no chance that the baby would be taken away. We felt happy and confident talking to Phil, grateful once again that we had found our way into Scott Roberts's Oklahoma network.

We had scheduled our sixth and final intrauterine insemination for the beginning of March. We considered canceling but decided to go ahead with it. It was somewhat perfunctory, as we now had all our attention focused on the baby in Oklahoma now entering his eighth month. Alexander was due around the end of April. At night and in the mornings, Bill and I would hold each other, put our heads together, and meditate, sending loving vibrations to him and Eileen. We bought books on baby care and called friends with older children to borrow a bassinet, baby clothes, and blankets. My friends planned a baby shower for the first weekend in April.

Now, my greatest regret about adopting was that I would not be able to breastfeed. I had heard that some adoptive mothers are able to produce milk, and, finally, through La Leche League, a group promoting breastfeeding, I found out about it. The process involves stimulating the nipples and breasts rather strenuously for at least a couple of months. You can use a breast pump (used by nursing mothers) as well as your hands. It requires commitment—up to an hour or two a day—and there is no promise it will work. Only a small percentage of women are actually able to stimulate lactation. It seemed like a major hassle and something I was unlikely to accomplish in three weeks. I also investigated a "breast bag" that enables you to store formula in a plastic bag next to the breast and feed the baby through a tube that runs to the nipple. The problem is that you have to start using it immediately after birth. We would probably not get Alexander until three or four days after he was born, and he would already be on a bottle. I also imagined trying to get hooked up in the breast bag gear on the airplane from Oklahoma. I began to let go of the breast-feeding fantasy, knowing that someday Alexander would come to enjoy the pleasures of a woman's breast in other ways.

When the delivery date was a few weeks away, I had Eileen on my mind constantly. Now I really began to worry about her changing her mind about giving up her baby. For the past two months, the real-life soap opera of the Baby M surrogacy case had been all over the news. We came to know the cast of characters: the anguished and emotional Mary Beth Whitehead, who refused to give up the child she gave birth to; and the Sterns, the distraught couple who believed the child to be theirs by virtue of Mr. Stern's sperm, a contract, and twenty thousand dollars. Although I could feel for Mary Beth Whitehead and knew how difficult it must be to give up the child she loved and nursed, it was hard for us not to identify with the Sterns and root for them to have custody of Baby M. At the time, our situation made us somewhat biased, and we did not think much about the obvious issues of sexism and classism in the case.

I wondered if Eileen was paying any attention to the Baby M case and if it was affecting her in any way. I wondered how she was feeling and whether she was afraid, anxious, or unhappy. I remembered the book *The Secret Life of the Unborn Child* and wondered how her state of mind would affect Alexander. Would he feel the effects of stress? Would he be an anxious and emotional child, prone to unhappiness? Had Eileen already separated herself from him emotionally so that he didn't feel loved? How would he feel during those two to three days after he was born when he would be in the hospital with no mother? I also wondered whether Eileen planned to see her baby after he was born. I wished I could talk with her, to let her know we were thinking about her and what she was going through, but I knew Scott wouldn't go for that. I did call him to see if sending her a letter might be a good idea. He said he'd give her the letter if that's what I wanted, but he strongly recommended against making any contact.

Even though I knew I probably wouldn't send it, I wrote to her anyway, just to have the feeling of communicating:

Dear Eileen,

I don't know if you will ever read this letter. Perhaps I am writing it more for myself than for you. But perhaps the caring that motivates my writing will find a way into your heart even if the words never reach you.

It is strange to be so intimately involved with someone I've never met. I will be the mother of your baby, whom we plan to call Alexander. Every day for many years I will look into eyes that are partially your eyes. I will hold a body made from your body. I will watch his face develop and wonder what you and his father look like.

I don't know what you went through in deciding that you didn't want any contact with us, but I am grateful for your decision. Bill and I had decided we didn't want an "open adoption." Instinctively, we felt we did not want to know our birth mother, did not want to risk involvement that might become entanglement. I know that it can work—biological and adoptive parents getting to know each other, staying in contact—but we just didn't want that responsibility. Perhaps it's for selfish reasons: to lessen any chance that you would want to take Alexander away from us; not being willing to share him with anyone; not wanting to be reminded that he came to us from someone else. But I don't feel our reasons are entirely selfish. I truly believe it is healthiest for you to say good-by to your baby forever—and not to be tempted to try to maintain a relationship with us or with him.

I don't expect for a minute that you will just forget about this little being you have lived with for nine months, but I hope that when he leaves you, you will not feel guilt, remorse, or regret. What I hope you will feel is a sense of fulfillment, of having given a precious gift to two other people, something we want more than anything in the world. We believe you are courageous in carrying our son and being willing to let him go. I don't know how much being Catholic had to do with your decision or what process you went through considering the other options of abortion or keeping the baby, but I know it must have been painful and difficult for you.

Never having been pregnant, I have never had to face the decision of an abortion. For that I am truly thankful. For even though I am not a Catholic and though I support a woman's right to choose to give birth or not, I doubt that I could ever have chosen to abort. When a life becomes a life is a mystery I doubt we will ever unravel, so each of us has to search our own heart for what is right. Thank you for having the courage and strength to bring our son into the world.

I hope and pray that Alexander's birth will be a completion for you—an experience you can feel complete about. I want you never to be haunted with doubt, guilt, or regret. I want you to appreciate your courage and your contribution to us and to the world. I want you to feel good about yourself and proud about your decision. I don't know what it will take for you to feel that way. Perhaps you already do. I hope you have been able to talk with your mother about your feelings or to get some sort of counseling that is supportive of you. I know it can't be easy.

I wonder, too, what you have thought about seeing the baby—whether you will want to see him, hold him, and say good-by—or whether you feel it would be easier on you not to see him. I am of two minds about it myself, thinking perhaps it might help your sense of completion to actually see him, but also that it might be difficult for you. I don't really know what I'd advise you, but I hope you give it some thought and feel good about your decision.

Bill and I think of you often. We pray that you are happy or at least not anxious and afraid. We wish we knew more about the father, what he looks like, his health history, etc. We appreciate that you've taken

care of yourself and don't smoke, drink, or do drugs.
We pray that Alexander will be robustly healthy and
that the birth will be as easy on you as possible.

I don't know if I will ever experience being pregnant or
giving birth. (You would probably tell me that's no
great loss right now.) We have no diagnosed reason for
our infertility, and perhaps, as *everyone* says, once we
adopt, I'll get pregnant. I would like that to happen.
But in deciding to adopt, I have had to let go of a lot
of ideas I had about having children. When we were
told you were brown-eyed and brunette, I was
disappointed. I wanted a blonde, blue-eyed baby, and
I wanted a little girl. I wanted a little me. What I had
to confront and realize is that my child is not me—that
children don't belong to us, even if we bear them. They
are themselves, unique and separate. I think I will be a
better mother having faced this fact. I will let
Alexander be who he is rather than what I want him
to be.

If you want to know about Alexander as he grows up,
Bill and I are happy to send you a letter and picture
once a year through Scott Roberts. If you don't want to
know about him, that's perfectly fine. When he's old
enough, we will be telling him about the beautiful
young woman who gave birth to him and how she
loved him so much that she gave him the best possible
home she could—with us.

Thank you, Eileen. We hope your life gets back to
normal soon, that you find success in whatever you
want to do, and that someday, when you're ready, you
have a wonderful family. Meanwhile, we will remain
intimate strangers, our lives linked in a powerful and
mysterious bond of love.

On Monday morning, about a week before the due date,
we received a call from Scott that on Sunday Eileen had

delivered a healthy, 8 pound, 6 ounce boy. The birth had been an easy one; she was in labor only a couple of hours. "He's a pretty-looking baby," Scott said, "and well-endowed, too. They're about to take him down to be circumcised right now."

"Scott!" I shrieked, "Get off the phone right now and call the hospital and stop them. We don't want him circumcised!" We couldn't believe we had forgotten to tell him we found this particular mutilation abhorrent and unnecessary. Twenty minutes later he called back and drawled, "Well, I couldn't get to 'em in time, but they said they could find it and sew it back on. There'll just be a kinda jagged scar...." It took us a minute to realize Scott was joking. He laughed uproariously as we got our hearts back up from our knees. We found out everything we could about Baby A, as we started to call him, thrilled that he had a high Apgar score (a standard measurement of a newborn's health) and that Scott kept telling us what a pretty baby he was. Then we called for reservations to Tulsa and made calls to all our family and friends. We stayed up half the night packing, preparing the "baby's room" (half of our bedroom) and dancing to the Talking Heads song about babies, "Up All Night."

For the next forty-eight hours we lived in a state of altered consciousness, so high we could hardly stand it. Early Tuesday morning, we flew to Oklahoma, studying Penelope Leach's book *Your Baby and Child* like we were cramming for an exam. We were met at the airport by Scott and then waited with him there for George and Doris, the couple who were adopting the half-Vietnamese baby. By coincidence, both mothers had delivered the same day, a first for Scott. The happiness of the occasion was marred a bit, however, because their baby was showing signs of a heart murmur. Another jolting surprise for Doris and George: Evidently, someone had made a mistake in reading the sonogram, and the baby they had thought was a girl was a boy. But dealing with a completely pink nursery and mounds of little dresses was the least of their worries. They were very concerned about the baby's health and not even sure they would take him if his heart was badly damaged. Talking with them and feeling their fear, I realized how unprepared we would have been for such an eventuality. We had assumed our son would be in perfect health, and he was, but what if it had been otherwise?

That afternoon, we were able to see our babies. For some reason known only to the hospital bureaucracy, we could not touch or hold them, we could only look through the glass of the nursery and see them in their little beds. We waited at the window a long time, joking nervously, wondering which of these swaddled bundles in various stages of sleep and crying would be coming home with us the next day. Finally, two beds were rolled to the window, and we knew which one was Alexander.

We pressed up against the glass and stared at him and cried. He was a beautiful baby! He wasn't wrinkled and mis-shapen but had a sweet, perfect face with Cupid lips and big blue eyes. He had hardly any hair on top, but it ringed the back of his head in Friar Tuck style. When we could take our eyes off Alexander, we also admired Justin (formerly Justine) who was smaller but also beautiful, with a mass of dark hair and softly sloped eyes. I had a strange feeling then, realizing this might have been our baby. In that moment, I knew that if he had been ours, I would have loved him just as much as I now loved Alexander.

What is the magic that creates this bond of love with a small, strange creature seen through a window? Perhaps it isn't really love; perhaps it's the fantasy of love. Perhaps it's helplessness that inspires caring or just an instinct that drives us to propagate our species. Whatever the source of the mystery, we knew we had just experienced "instant bonding." We had literally fallen in love at first sight, and our lives would never be the same.

Through our tears of joy, we inquired about Eileen, and Scott told us she had left the hospital the day before. She was in good spirits, he said, grateful that the birth had been an easy one. She had said she was glad the baby had come early, since she would have more time to lose weight before her high school graduation. We knew that Eileen might not start really feeling what had happened for several days, but we were relieved that now she seemed to be looking forward to moving on with her life.

Waiting the twenty hours until we could pick up our boy from the hospital was difficult but made as enjoyable as possible by Scott and his wonderful wife, Margaret. Generous far beyond the call of duty, they took the four of us out to dinner at one of Tulsa's best restaurants, where Scott flirted mercilessly with the waitresses and joked with all the other "good ol' boys." My Southern accent was warmed up and well oiled by a few glasses of wine, and I felt right at home. George and Doris functioned well under the strain. They were waiting for tests that would be done in the morning and didn't want to talk much about how they were feeling, but they did their best to join in the party atmosphere. We did our best not to act too completely ecstatic and not to talk too much about Alexander.

By morning, they had good news. Justin's heart murmur was almost gone. The doctor wanted him to stay in the hospital a few days for observation, but the prognosis was excellent —he would likely suffer no ill effects from it. We all celebrated at breakfast, and then Bill and Scott and I were off for a whirlwind morning. First we met the judge in his chambers; he solemnly warned us that we could not return the child at age 2 or when he became a teenager. Then we spent an hour at the county courthouse signing and stamping a pile of papers two inches high, Scott complaining all the time about California's requiring sixteen different consent forms from the birth mother. Finally, the papers were filed, and we were off to the hospital to wait once again for the bureaucratic gears to turn out our baby.

As it happened, the hospital would not turn the baby over directly to us, even though we were now the legal guardians. This particular hospital had a fundamentalist orientation and was not too keen on private adoption. They had their own home for "wayward girls" and turned the babies over to the county agency to be placed with appropriately religious families. As we waited in the lobby, a woman hospital volunteer accosted us to inquire about our religion, and soon she and Bill were in a heated theological debate. I just wanted to get Alexander and get out of there. Finally, we were told they would bring him to Scott's car. A few minutes later, out by the car, a stonefaced nurse carrying a blue bundle brushed past us without so much as a glance. She opened the car door, handed the baby to Scott, and then locked the door as she closed it. It was quite clear how this hospital felt about us.

But from that moment on, nothing mattered but this sweet face swaddled in baby blankets. As we ogled our boy in the back seat, Scott drove us to his home, where he and Margaret helped us feed and change him and get ourselves ready for the trip. Somehow, we made it to the airport and onto a plane, through another airport, and onto another plane, all the while staring in ecstasy at our son, passing him gently back and forth between us. A woman passenger sitting across the aisle from us leaned over to tell us, "They're not as fragile as they seem. Don't worry, he won't break." Baby A slept his way across the country and even through dinner at a restaurant with our friends Katherine and Vern. Finally, we made it home to our little house—a family at last.

Chapter Six

Life With Baby

*B*ooks about infertility usually end when life with baby begins. Talking about babies just doesn't seem appropriate, perhaps for fear that dwelling on the joys of parenthood will just cause pain for the prefertile reader—like attending a baby shower. I sincerely hope that will not be the case here. For I continue our story not to make you uncomfortable, but rather to encourage you onward to the joy that awaits you. Becoming a family does not mean the pain of infertility goes away, but for us the happiness and fulfillment of at last having a child completely overwhelmed it. Waiting for baby was over, and we were facing new issues now—the day-to-day care of our new little being.

Alexander, our cherub-cheeked, Cupid-lipped beauty, made us ecstatically happy. He was a perfect baby—good-natured, cheerful, and healthy. He cried, of course, but he was easily comforted. He enthralled our friends and family and kept us saying to each other, "I don't think we could have made one better!" We loved him more than we could imagine loving anyone, and it made absolutely no difference that he did not come from our genes or my womb. In fact, we watched with curiosity and anticipation for signs of what he would look like. Would he surpass Bill's and my genetic flaws? (We both have short legs and long noses and wished him the opposite.) When would he ever get hair on the top of his head? Would his eyes stay blue like mine or turn hazel like Bill's? Would he keep those adorable dimples and those sweet bow lips? Although I was curious, I was still glad that we had not seen a picture of Eileen and did not know what he was supposed to look like. There was no image for him to fit; he just became more and more beautiful—an angel, our angel.

Bill was thrilled to be a father, and he turned out to be my image of the perfect daddy—gentle, playful, adoring, and willing to clean up even the messiest diaper. He was also strong and consistent, able to take charge when I panicked. (The first night, Alexander started throwing up, and I was so upset I started throwing up. Bill ministered to both of us and calmed us both down.) He participated fully in the night-to-night care, as we traded off getting up for feedings—a major blessing of bottle feeding. Together we inhabited the Twilight Zone of constantly interrupted sleep (they torture people that way, you know), but Bill had the ability to fall asleep any time and just about anywhere. Frequently I'd find him sprawled on the living room floor or napping on the front seat of his truck in front of the house. For the first time in my life, I was able to take naps during the day, though most of the time I would just lie and look at Baby A swaddled next to me.

In those first few weeks, our lives were completely focused on Alexander. We worried mainly about bottles (thank God for microwave ovens in the middle of the night) and nipples (boiling them until no microbe could possibly survive). We talked mainly about baby poop (when, how much, and what color) and schedules (when did you feed him last? when do you think he'll go down again?). We argued the value of letting him cry (but never letting him do so for more than five minutes) and the pros and cons of pacifiers. On the advice of the doctor ("try not to give it to him or he'll get hooked"), I did without a pacifier for a couple of weeks. Then, during one predawn crying jag, when Alexander was inconsolable with the bottle and I was exhausted and desperate, I somehow managed to put my breast in his mouth. Immediately, he started sucking ferociously and stopped crying. This would have been great except that it was excruciatingly painful. Untrained nipples are not meant for this kind of treatment! When I couldn't stand it anymore, I substituted the Nuk pacifier. That night, I discovered their magic, and *I* was hooked.

During this time, we didn't worry much about Eileen changing her mind, although we did feel some relief after ten days had passed and she could no longer petition to get the baby back in Oklahoma. We knew it was highly unlikely she would come to California to file suit. When we thought of Eileen, it was not with fear but with the deepest gratitude. She had given us the greatest gift anyone could give, and we were even a little sad that we hadn't gotten to know her and couldn't thank her, even though we couldn't have thanked her enough. I had the sense that she might be more in touch now with her loss, and though I couldn't speak to her, I said prayers that she was happy and at peace with herself.

A couple of weeks after Alexander was born, the *Life* photographer returned for shots of the three of us. It seems they were considering putting us on the cover of the issue about infertility. We were thrilled, but Baby A couldn't have cared less. He insisted on snoozing through the session, blinking wildly when the flash went off and then falling back to sleep. In the end, *Life* didn't use any of the shots. Instead, on the cover of the June 1987 issue, entitled "The Try-Everything World of Baby-Craving," was a gorgeous 1-year-old, the world's first "host womb" baby. Although our pictures illustrated the cover story, we were not really the focus of the story, and we were somewhat disappointed. Still, it was fun to have people in the grocery checkout line say, "Didn't I just see your picture in *Life* magazine?"

When the issue came out, we began our career as the unofficial "infertile couple of the year." Bill and I appeared on local television a couple of times and then received a call from "The CBS Morning Program." They wanted to fly us to New York for an appearance in July. We would be talking about infertility with host Mariette Hartley and a fertility specialist. The trip turned out to be great fun, even though our few days in New York coincided with the summer's worst heat wave. Alexander traveled like a champ, staying quiet on the plane and mostly sleeping as we wheeled him around stores, restaurants, and museums. He seemed unfazed by the 95 degree heat and the 95 percent humidity. (Perhaps it was his Oklahoma blood.) The hotel found a sweet elderly Southern woman, Mary Laura, to baby-sit for us while we did the town at night. Living in a hotel with a baby was great fun: rolling around with him on the king-size bed, bathing him in the sink, ordering formula from room service.

The appearance on CBS went well. We were nervous but fairly articulate, trying to tell about the most difficult years of our lives in a five-minute time slot. Luckily, we didn't know Alexander was screaming his head off in the "green room." TV producers, even female ones, don't know what to do with howling babies. After New York, we were able to go to North Carolina to show him off to my family.

At home again, Baby A did change our lives. We had friends over more often than we went out and rented movies months old to watch on video (another technological blessing for new parents—the VCR). But he really didn't slow us down too much. The great thing about a little guy is that he is so portable. We took him almost everywhere—to parties and restaurants, even on a sailing outing—but we never took him to movies (not having a breast handy when he cried did have its disadvantages).

At two and half months, we took him to a picnic for Scott Roberts's adoptive families. This was not the biannual event with Scott and Margaret, but a wonderful get-together for the families to stay in touch with each other. We proudly showed off our boy and became reacquainted with the folks we'd met when we were "expecting." We particularly wanted Alexander to meet his nursery buddy, Justin. He was a completely healthy, beautiful baby, who, like almost all of the kids there, looked just like his parents.

At the picnic, the couples who lived in Marin County warned us about the social worker who would be visiting us. She was, we were told, an advocate of open adoption who would grill us about why we hadn't met the birth mother, and perhaps even want to try to contact her. They had found her cold and aloof, and on occasion, they had heard, she had tried to delay adoptions. We were getting a little nervous about our interview, due to happen soon, but when our call came from the Social Services Department, it was not from a woman, but from a man. He was substituting for the regular worker while she was on maternity leave and would be sending us forms to fill out. Then he said he'd try to visit us as soon as possible.

The adoption questionnaire was truly bizarre. We were asked all manner of personal questions, including when we had first had sex and how we felt about it. We were asked about our familial relationships, our past therapy experience, and our philosophy of life. The kicker, of course, was "Why do you want to have children?" What was the right answer? Why did they ask us this? Why didn't they ask this of everyone who got a marriage license? We considered answering some of the questions NOYB—None of Your Business—but figured this was a game we had better play along with.

The day of our social worker's visit, I cleaned the house scrupulously and Bill took off from work. We waited around nervously for forty-five minutes before I called his office to find him there. He had written down a different date. How about next week? When he did finally come to see us, our fears dissipated quickly. Barry was a tall, handsome young man who listened to us, drew us out with questions, and was obviously supportive of our adoption. We had lucked out once again.

Our conversation with Barry focused a good bit on how we would deal with adoption issues—when and how would we tell Alexander and others about his being adopted. To both of us, the issue of adoption seemed very matter-of-fact. From the beginning, we had been quite open about it, finding ourselves telling total strangers in the grocery store or in restaurants or at the airport. Finally having been admitted to the sorority of women with baby-filled grocery carts, I stopped often in the aisles to talk to other new mothers and exclaim over their babies: "Isn't she beautiful! How old is she? Is she sleeping through the night?" Discussions ensued, and I watched as their eyes fell on Alexander and then on my flat belly and small breasts. I knew the unasked question forming in their minds, "How did she lose that weight so fast?" I didn't let them wonder long. "Yes, he's adorable. We adopted him three months ago." Bill, too, liked to tell people Alexander was adopted, and sometimes we almost bragged about it, I suppose because we wanted to break people's stereotypic view of adoption as something to be hidden. I guess we also wanted people to know that there were successful adoptions.

After a while, though, we became a bit more circumspect, not hiding but not volunteering the information so easily. Often, when we told our story, people would half-joke that we'd "done it the easy way." Ha. And almost invariably their comment would be, "You watch, now you'll get pregnant." This was perhaps the most annoying response to our adoption, and

it came from almost everyone we knew, close friends and
family as well as acquaintances. *Everyone*, it seemed, knew
someone who had adopted and a few months later got pregnant. It was one of the great lingering myths about adoption
that seemed to have permeated our society, despite the Stan-
ford University study that showed the same rate of pregnancy
for adoptive couples as for infertile couples who did not
adopt—about 5 percent.

We just didn't know how to explain to people that it was
an inappropriate response, reflecting the old notion that all
you need to do is "relax" to get pregnant. It also in some small
way devalued the child you had, as if he or she was but a
stepping stone to the "real thing." I knew people didn't mean
it that way, but it bugged us. After the twentieth story of an
adoption-spawned pregnancy, we'd just smile and say, "Well,
we hope that will happen."

But truly, we didn't want it to happen—not for many
months, anyway. We had our hands completely full with one
of these creatures. I shuddered at how I once thought it would
be great to have twins. Still, we didn't use birth control, but
then again, it wasn't really necessary. The really big changes
in your life once baby arrives are no sleep and *no sex*. Even
though I was not recovering from the exhaustion of childbirth,
I was hardly in a romantic frame of mind, and living in the
Twilight Zone didn't enhance our sex life. Luckily, Bill felt the
same way, so we both just cuddled and focused our adoration
on our little bundle in blue. We knew someday we would
make love again. . . .

Life with Alexander was easier and more fun than I could
ever have imagined—in part because he was such a great baby
and certainly because I was so ready to have a child. I had
no regrets at all about cutting way back on my work, putting
away my dresses, suits, and high heels and hanging out at
home in sweat suits with no make-up on. Instead of running
around all the time, I was doing a lot of sitting and rocking

in my big stuffed rocking chair. Sitting there with babe in arms staring out at sunlit leaves and all varieties of sky, I felt content in a way I had never felt before. My lifelong drive to achieve, to be somebody, to have some impact on the world, seemed to have at last been satisfied. Achieving motherhood, being a parent, and being responsible for the growth of another human being felt very significant—as important as ending world hunger or stopping the nuclear arms race. For the first time in my life, I felt relaxed at the core of my being. My friends commented on how different my energy felt. I laughed and said that I was just exhausted, but I knew there was more to it than that. Some fundamental need had at last been met, and I was fully and completely *happy*.

Like many other women who have babies so late in life, I guess I became a "born again" mother, utterly enthusiastic about the adventure of raising a child. I had to catch myself with mothers who told me they were going back to work full-time a few months or a year after their child's birth. "Oh, how terrible" I wanted to say, forgetting that some women are not so enamored of motherhood. Of course, there are many who are but who have to work for financial reasons, and now I began to feel deeply for their dilemma. Issues like parental leave and childcare that I had never paid much attention to began to concern me. All of a sudden, I had joined a new interest group. I was now a part of the populace for whom "family" issues would come to dominate the political and social agenda.

Perhaps it is only when you live with a baby day to day and see how completely helpless he is, how his very being is shaped by the nature and consistency of the care he receives, that you realize how crucial family life is for the development of our psyches and, consequently, our society. As I witnessed our son settling into this new life, knowing he would be held, comforted, fed, and loved, I could not help but think with horror of the infants and children who were subjected to neglect and abuse. At times, when Alexander's wailing turned into a contented cooing the second the bottle reached his mouth, I could feel the pain of a mother who had no milk, no food to feed her crying child, and I cried. Life with baby is lived in the very heart of what it means to be human.

Loving this child so completely and so deeply, I began to feel very vulnerable and at times afraid. What if something should happen to him? When a woman in my dance exercise class told me about her son's having died of SIDS—Sudden Infant Death syndrome—I became almost paranoid about it. The cause of these infant deaths is completely unknown, and they usually occur among baby boys while they are sleeping. If Alexander took an especially long nap during the day, I'd find myself checking on him to make sure he was breathing, and at night sometimes I would get up and touch him just to feel him warm and stirring. I could not imagine how I could cope with losing our son. I thought of all the possible dangers and tried, without being overprotective, to be aware of anything that might happen. Even though we knew that Eileen could not take Alexander from us now, we felt happy and relieved the day our adoption was final.

As Alexander inhabited our home and our hearts, he felt so completely ours that we didn't think much about issues of adoption—when, how, and what we would tell him about his birth situation and what impact being adopted would have on his psyche. That would all come in time. We did think about the blessings of adoption, particularly the feeling we had that we would never take this child for granted. As much as we loved him as our own son, we knew that we did not "own" this being. We felt we might even have an advantage over biological parents, who may find it easier to forget that children are not their possessions, but separate people whose lives they help shape but should not dominate. We hoped we would always keep the perspective of serving as a guide for our son, remembering the words of Kahlil Gibran's *The Prophet*:

> *Your children are not your children.*
> *They are the sons and daughters of Life's longing for*
> *itself.*
> *They come through you but not from you,*
> *And though they are with you yet they belong not to*
> *you.**

We had been given the greatest gift anyone could receive, but this gift of life was ours only to love and nurture. We were blessed and inspired by this sacred trust.

---

*Kahlil Gibran, *The Prophet*. New York (Alfred A. Knopf, 1923).

Part Two

❧

Introduction

*I*t is my hope not only that our story has encouraged you in your journey through the painful process of infertility, but that it has also given you the sense that what awaits you at the end of your long ordeal is truly worth it. Obviously, our story is not a typical one. In fact, there is no "typical" infertile couple and no typical adoption. Some of what Bill and I went through may feel relevant to you and some may not. Ours is but one small success story intended to offer some hope. I began this book intending that our story and those of people we have come to know could cover many of the issues involved in waiting for baby, but as our story came to a close, I found there was more I wanted to say. There is much information that I did not have during our infertility and adoption, and there are many ideas and perspectives that have become clear to me only at the end of our journey.

Having talked with dozens of prefertile and infertile cou-

ples, several fertility specialists, and many adoptive parents
and adoption counselors over the past three years, I feel in a
position to offer some straightforward advice that I hope will
support you in your quest to have a baby. My advice is aimed
at helping you to keep moving through what I call "the infertility maze," that maddening, frustrating labyrinth of medical
and emotional problems that many of us spend years trying
to escape from.

For those of us who want children more than anything
else in life, our quest to make a baby can easily become an
obsession, crowding out other aspects of our lives and cloud-
ing our good judgment. Emotionally, we are plagued by
self-doubt, sometimes chronic depression, and often marital
problems. Socially, we feel left out of the world of families
and children, and our career motivation generally gets lost in
the shuffle. Medically, we look to an area of treatment that is
in its infancy, and we expect it to work miracles for us. It has
been said that infertility patients are surpassed only by ter-
minal cancer patients in their willingness to undergo difficult,
expensive procedures with low rates of success.

Making it through the maze with your sanity, finances,
and relationships relatively unscathed requires both emotional
sensitivity and rational decision making. The next chapter
offers some suggestions about how to take care of yourself
and your relationships, how to deal effectively with doctors,
and how to approach decisions about medical treatment as
well as other options for having or not having children. I hope
it will inform, encourage, and motivate you in your journey.

Since many of you may decide to seek your family
through adoption, in chapter 8 I offer an overview of this
institution that is going through such enormous change now.
As you may have surmised, our wonderful experience with
Scott Roberts, the Oklahoma Stork, is not a common one for
adoptive parents. Having found such a quick, easy, and successful path toward adopting Alexander, Bill and I were bliss-

fully unaware of the web of complexities woven around adoption for most couples.

When we first started thinking about it, we saw adoption as a situation in which everyone wins. We knew we would be great parents. We knew we could give a child more than could an unwed mother who had not yet experienced life and who would probably find having a young child a great burden. We believed we would be giving some young person a gift almost as great as the one we would receive—the freedom to grow and develop without the responsibility of raising a small child.

Without thinking much about it, we knew that we would always be open with our child about his birth circumstances, and we were sure that there would be no stigma or damaging psychological effect from being adopted. We found it hard to imagine that in our liberal community our child would ever be taunted by other children because of his adoptive status. We knew that adopted children sometimes wanted to find their biological parents, especially their birth mothers, but we assumed their desire stemmed either from simple curiosity or from the fact that they found their childhood and their relationship with their adoptive parents lacking in some way. We, of course, would be such great parents that our child would have little concern about his biological roots—curiosity, perhaps, but no driving need to find or know his "real parents." If he did want to know, we would support him in finding his birth mother at some appropriate age.

We knew that private adoption was risky, that sometimes birth parents changed their minds, but we also knew we had no alternative. Given the strictures and biases of adoption agencies, unless we wanted to take a handicapped child or were willing to wait perhaps years for a foreign adoption or were blessed with the miracle of pregnancy, this was the only way we would ever have a baby.

We knew about open adoption but suffered from the

same fear and skepticism most would-be adopters have about an approach that on the surface seemed to value and protect the birth parents over the adoptive parents-to-be. We assumed that any contact with us or the child would only complicate the birth mother's life and make it more difficult for her to let go, forget, and move on. We were completely unaware of the problems of women who have given up babies and of the problems that many people see in the adoptive family— unhappy, maladjusted children and nervous, overprotective parents.

Once we had Alexander in our lives and knew he was ours, we figured we were among the luckiest people on the planet, especially since we believed that Scott Roberts would also help us find a second baby when the time was right. We would have our complete family, and that would be that. I doubt we would have thought much more about adoption had I not undertaken writing this book. Perhaps we could have remained ignorant of all the sticky issues surrounding adoption and been no worse off for it. Perhaps not.

If you think you'll be moving in the adoption direction, you may need a good deal more information than we had, and you may need to examine your own attitudes and fears more closely than we did. There are a number of important questions to be considered in the process of adopting, and understanding them will help you in your decision to adopt as well as enhance your chances for success if you do.

Whatever path you take, I hope the following two chapters are useful to you in determining the future of your family life.

Chapter Seven

❦

Moving Through the Infertility Maze

*E*ach individual and couple has their own unique experience of waiting for baby, depending on where they are in the process and who they are as people. But all of us who face a period of infertility share a sense of having entered strange and unknown territory. Babies are supposed to happen naturally, after all. Procreation is not something you are supposed to have to think about or figure out, much less pay other people for. Reluctantly, we acknowledge that "doing what comes naturally" isn't working, and we begin an odyssey that takes us into a strange new land of doctors, treatments, emotions, and decisions.

The process of discovering, treating, and resolving infertility is like a journey through an elaborate maze, a labyrinth of medical, emotional, and financial choices with no clear path to a happy ending. The maze itself is difficult enough, but there are two of you trying to negotiate this journey, three or more

if you count doctors and others who want to give you advice.
At first, there is the surprise (and sometimes, unfortunately,
the shame) that you are stuck some place you don't want to
be. Then come the brave, dogged attempts to find a way out.
A seemingly hopeful turn dead ends. You try again. Another
dead end, and another, and another. You find yourself dou-
bling back through old territory, confused about where you've
been and where you're going. You get separated from your
partner, or he or she doesn't want to take the same route or
move as fast as you do. You are reunited, feeling confident
of a particular path, but then you get nowhere. The maze does
have an end point, although it's not the same for everyone.
You find it in your own way in your own time, and it can be
a joyous resolution, a sad resignation, or simply a time-out for
R & R before jumping in again.

As I have come to know more and more prefertile couples,
I am almost thankful that I was already forty years old when
I confronted our infertility. I knew I had a discrete amount
of time, hopefully at least five years, in which I could hope for
childbearing. And I was certain that I wanted to have children
and would, even if it meant adopting. But I didn't want to
become a mother when my friends were becoming grandparents. I wanted to move and move fast. It was two and a half
years from the time Bill and I started Trying until we brought
Alexander home with us.

Not all prefertile couples need or want to move that fast.
Some couples in their twenties and early thirties with other
priorities competing with childrearing can afford a more lei-
surely wait and a slower pace of fertility treatment. But for
some, age is irrelevant. You may want a baby and want it now,
and whether you are 25, 35, or 45 makes no difference. Whatever your timetable, however, no one wants to get stuck in the
fertility maze. It is difficult, frustrating, time-consuming, and
expensive, not to mention emotionally painful, draining, and
sometimes agonizing. It tests your ability to deal with your

emotions, your communication and support as a couple, and your relationships with other people—friends and family as well as medical professionals.

To keep moving through the infertility labyrinth requires sensitivity, stamina, and perseverance. It calls on you to learn to take care of yourself emotionally, to move through self-blame and self-pity and find strength in yourself and your relationship. It also demands that you educate yourself, take responsibility for your treatment, and make difficult choices. Most important, it challenges you to keep true to your vision that you *will* have a family.

The most difficult part of navigating the infertility maze is allowing yourself to experience, express, and move through the emotional states that result from being on the seesaw of constant hope and disappointment. Recycling monthly through these emotions, it is easy to get stuck either nurturing false hopes for success or spiraling down into constant expectations of failure. Whether those feelings are rational and justified by the circumstances or whether they are irrational, stemming from myths and misperceptions, they demand attention and resolution.

Infertility expert Barbara Eck Menning, the founder of RESOLVE and author of the book *Infertility: A Guide for the Childless Couple*, has identified the major emotional states most couples go through in trying to resolve their infertility. She found that infertile couples experience feelings of denial, anger, guilt, depression, and grief. While she characterizes these feelings as successive emotional stages, she points out that they do not necessarily represent a linear process. Couples and individuals may move back and forth between stages at different times.

Looking back at Bill's and my experience over two and a half years, the stages reflect pretty accurately our emotions and our process of resolution. What I think helped us stay fairly positive during our years of Trying was that we were able to let our feelings flow, that we didn't get stuck in any one phase too long. It is when emotions are blocked and remain unexperienced and unexpressed that they start to eat away at your energy, your self-esteem, your self-confidence, and your relationship. Learning to move in and out of various emotional states is crucial to moving through the infertility maze.

Denial, usually the first reaction to infertility, is initially useful, giving you time to absorb what is happening and develop ways of coping. Accepting that you have fertility problems is a gradual process, but at some point you and your partner have to admit that it's time to pursue a course of action. If you get stuck denying there is a problem, you may not seek appropriate treatment or may feel isolated and alone, unable to get the emotional support you need.

When you do acknowledge that something is wrong, you may find yourself feeling angry and resentful. Why me? Why us? It's not fair! Anger is an emotion many people have difficulty feeling and even more difficulty expressing. It's not nice to be angry. If we do let ourselves feel it, we think we have to be angry at someone, so we turn our feelings of frustration and rage in on ourselves or out on other people. Spouses are the closest at hand, of course, but doctors, nurses, bosses, and fertile family and friends are also likely candidates. Repressed anger or anger turned inward leads to feelings of depression and apathy; turned outward, it can be inappropriate and hurtful. Moving through anger in a healthy way first of all means believing it is okay to be angry—at a specific person or situation or at everyone and everything. If you can't be specific in expressing anger at someone, you need to find some appropriate way to release the energy—by hitting a pillow, throwing something expendable, or yelling while you're alone at home or driving in your car. Getting good and angry is often refreshing and doesn't have to be directed at any one or any thing in particular.

Guilt, I've always heard it said, is a "useless emotion," I guess because it is something we tend to wallow in. It rarely moves us in any direction. It goes right along with shame and blame, our attempts to pass judgment on ourselves and others. Whether or not you can hold yourself responsible in some way for your infertility—say you chose the wrong type of birth control or you made a hasty decision to have a vasectomy—or whether it's clearly your spouse's problem and not yours, blame, shame, and guilt do nothing but demoralize. Letting go of guilt and blame means simply forgiving yourself or your partner. Sometimes it is not easy, and it may not happen just by saying, "I forgive you, I forgive myself" once or twice. You may need to draw on forgiveness whenever the feelings come up in order to continue the healing process.

As is apparent in our story, experiencing and expressing grief are an unavoidable part of resolving infertility. Feeling sad and crying are very normal reactions to not being able to have the child you want, but often people find it difficult to acknowledge their feelings of grief and to give themselves permission to let them out. The "loss" of an unconceived child is an abstraction to most people. Mourning such an invisible loss can be difficult, and friends and family may offer little consolation or support.

We also get stuck in grief by not allowing its full expression. We fear that if we do "let it all out," we will lose control, fall apart and, like Humpty Dumpty, never get ourselves back together again. It is a lesson I seem to have to learn over and over again—how good it feels to "have a good cry." It takes an enormous amount of energy to hold back tears, and yet it is almost instinctive to try not to cry. It may be easier for women than for men, but all of us resist our sadness and forget how our tears seem to cleanse our souls. Often, when I've thought I could cry all day or all night, five minutes of sobbing will release and renew.

It is important to know that grief does not last forever.

It runs its course and leaves us in a state of acceptance, a place from which we can make decisions and move on. Acceptance may come more easily for couples who have a specific diagnosis and have exhausted their treatment opportunities. But with so many new treatment technologies developing, there is always the tendency to want to try the next thing and the next and the next. For couples like Bill and me, who suffer from unexplained infertility, acceptance is also difficult. There's no known reason why it couldn't happen any month now. Acceptance does not mean "giving up," however. Rather, it is accepting the situation you are in ("We don't know if it will ever happen") and moving on from there.

Part of moving successfully through the emotional turmoil is managing the impact of infertility on your relationship. Like any major adversity in life, infertility can bring couples closer together or pull them apart. I doubt that many truly happy marriages are destroyed by the inability to have a child, but infertility can become the issue around which other problems coalesce—a scapegoat, as it were, for other, unexpressed dissatisfactions. The stress of waiting for baby can take its toll even on the happiest couples, creating pressures and resentments that would not ordinarily surface. How you cope with those problems can strain a marriage but can also strengthen it.

In facing a situation we found we had no control over, Bill and I pulled together, feeling the power of our partnership. We found we had to examine our life's goals and be clearer and more purposeful about pursuing what we wanted. We learned about each other's dreams and fears and came to a deeper understanding of how to empathize with and support each other. We were able to read each other's hearts, grieve together, and give each other comfort and encouragement.

Most of the prefertile couples I have known also feel that the experience strengthened their relationship. Not that they would wish it on anyone, but it gave them an opportunity to grow together. This perspective may be useful when you find yourselves stuck in the infertility maze. And you are most apt to get stuck when you and your partner are out of sync in your feelings about what you're doing—or not doing. It's frightening and depressing to find yourself alone all of a sudden, with the partner you counted on lagging behind or taking off ahead of you. Sometimes you may be moving along with such dogged determination that you don't even notice he or she is no longer beside you. You may be so absorbed in your own feelings that you don't even notice your partner's reluctance or his or her eagerness to move faster than you want to. You may not recognize you're out of sync until a crisis of some sort brings you to a screeching halt.

While there are certainly exceptions, in most instances it is the man who drags his feet. The woman usually takes the lead through the infertility labyrinth. We women are the ones pushing for action and often pulling our mates along. Having children is a crucial part of who we are as females; it is a purpose of our existence and a basic element of our self-concept. Even a career woman who has put a great deal of energy into her work finds it difficult to exclude mothering from her life's agenda. We women are usually the ones to bear the brunt of the treatment grind and the monthly bleeding away of hopes and dreams. We may find ourselves resenting our men, blaming them for "not really caring," "not being enthusiastic about the treatment," "not wanting to make decisions."

While men may feel as deeply as we do the pain of longing for children, they are generally able to let go of it more easily and focus their attention on work and career. Men are "doers"; they find it difficult to feel helpless and out of control. In response to frustration, a man is more likely to withdraw, to try to be "rational," and to downplay his emotions in order to protect his partner. Bill would often not express his feelings of disappointment and despair, and when I'd challenge him for not caring enough, he'd tell me, "Honey, I feel I have to be strong so I can support you. What would happen if we were both basket cases?"

In addition to clamming up emotionally at home, it is generally difficult for men to talk about their procreation problems with other men. It's hard to imagine a guy at a bar saying to his buddy, "Say, did I tell you about this problem I have with my sperm count?" or calling up a friend in tears to tell him, "Mary just started her period today." But whether it is expressed as openly or as easily, men do carry their portion of the infertility burden, particularly with regard to sexuality and the sexual relationship.

For men who know that the fertility problem is theirs, there may be the emotional effect of the connection between fertility and virility. Even though it isn't rational, there is the psychological stigma of "not being a real man," of "shooting blanks," or of feeling impotent. Sometimes that feeling can be manifested in actual sexual dysfunction, particularly given the necessity of sex on demand at "that time of the month." Unlike their partners, men can't fake sexual arousal. Command sexual performances aren't always successful, and premature ejaculation or even impotence can result from the pressure. Even producing a sperm sample can be difficult and embarrassing. Women need to keep in mind what it would feel like to be told to "have an orgasm in five minutes here in the doctor's office."

Women, too, can experience sexual problems: sometimes the inability to have orgasms but usually the lack of desire for sex. So much attention goes into the purposeful aspects of procreation that sex for sex's sake is almost forgotten. Sometimes both partners try to put off sex for days or weeks until the right time, not realizing that men only need one or two days to recover their sperm count. Once I asked Bill to abstain from orgasm for almost two weeks in order to "save up sperm," but I think partly I just wanted to avoid intercourse. He often felt the same way.

Navigating the sexual seas takes sensitivity and a sense of humor. It is important to remember that it is normal for sexual problems to come up during prefertility and that they are usually transient. You can help them move along by giving yourself and your partner a break—both figuratively and literally. Give yourselves permission not to have sex and instead try cuddling, giving each other a massage, or otherwise pleasuring each other. Perhaps take a vacation from Trying now and then and let spontaneity be the source of your sexual encounters. Throw the thermometer out the window, tear up the chart, and pretend you are newlyweds again. And for God's sake, let yourselves laugh. Granted, I haven't heard any great infertility jokes, but for each of us there are absurd situations that you can respond to only with a sense of humor.

Dealing with sexual misconnections and dysfunctions is part of the overall challenge of keeping infertility from taking over your relationship. The key, of course, is to keep communicating and not to lose each other in the maze. It's one thing to know that communication is the answer to all relationship problems; it's another to actually communicate effectively. The problem among infertile couples is often that the women communicate too much and the men too little. In many cases, women talk constantly about the problem—the frustrations of the temperature chart, the trials of treatment, the small, everyday agonies of being infertile in a fertile world. Many men turn off to the topic, preferring not to have talk about it again and again, especially since there's nothing they can *do* about it. Sometimes, of course, the problem is the other way around, but in either case you need to find ways to share your feelings without letting them take over your life.

If you find yourself out of sync with your mate and unable to communicate effectively, you may want to seek some kind of counseling or join a RESOLVE support group. Sometimes group sessions are the first occasion men have to talk to other men, and couples get to see how other couples handle their problems. You can also impose some objectivity on your own day-to-day communication by focusing your infertility conversations. RESOLVE groups often suggest that you set a specific period of time each day, say ten minutes, for each of you to share your feelings and frustrations. Each person must talk, but then you must put the issue aside and focus on other aspects of your life.

Dealing with your loving partner may be easier than dealing with the ignorance or insensitivity of others in your life. Of course, you don't have to broadcast your infertility nationwide as Bill and I did, but the topic will come up. "Do you two have any kids?" "When are you guys going to start a family?" "Are you pregnant yet?" Friends, family members, coworkers, or acquaintances who have no experience with infertility and its pain can sometimes say very stupid and hurtful things. When yet another person tells you to "relax and don't try so hard," you may be tempted just to slug him or her and vow never to mention your problem again. It's okay not to talk to people you don't care about, but with folks close to you, it's important that you share your feelings and also that you educate them about how to respond to you appropriately. Let people know that they don't have to *do* anything but just *be* there for you. Tell them that, rather than giving you more advice or simplistic reassurance, you want them just to understand and accept what you're feeling, whether it's anger, hurt, or sadness. I really appreciated my friend who said simply, "I know how much you want to have a baby and how difficult it must be. Just let me know what you're feeling and I'll always try to support you." She didn't try to "fix" me or cheer me up but just let me cry on her shoulder when I needed to.

It helps, also, to seek out other couples who are waiting

for baby. More and more infertile couples are coming out of the closet and finding each other. Among your fellow prefertiles you will find not only emotional and spiritual support, but also valuable information about doctors and procedures. Almost everyone who becomes involved with RESOLVE, the national organization for infertile couples, reports how important it is no longer to feel isolated and alone with the problem. Knowing that one in six couples has this trouble, it's difficult to feel you are being singled out for punishment by God.

Talking to other couples may help you deal with some of the impact of infertility on your job or career. While most men find that fertility problems do not affect their work, women often find that pursuing pregnancy is like taking on a new job—with all the attendant demands and stress. If you are already working for a living, holding down two jobs can be truly harrowing. How to explain all those times you have to leave work for a "doctor's appointment"? It generally feels best to tell the truth about what you are going through, but some women feel if they tell their employers they are trying to get pregnant, their jobs or future advancement will be jeopardized. More often, the problem at work is lack of motivation, just not having the focus or the energy to be creative, work long hours, or take on new responsibilities. At times it may be feelings of depression distracting you; at other times it may be high hopes—why go for it if you'll soon be on maternity leave?

For people whose jobs bring them in touch daily with children or pregnant women, going to work can be particularly difficult. Obviously, working in a day-care center and selling maternity clothes aren't the best choices for prefertiles, but all jobs have their challenges—such as dealing with co-workers who brag about their kids or attending yet another office baby shower. Nevertheless, work can also be a haven from the waiting-for-baby blues, giving you a place to focus your energy and providing opportunities for self-expression and pride of accomplishment. Your work may be the one area in your life where you feel you have some power and control, and you may be lucky enough to have co-workers who give you support and nurturing.

There is no one prescription for how to integrate your career with the emotional and time demands of moving through the infertility maze. The only advice I can give is to go easy on yourself. Keep in mind that you are going through a major life crisis and you cannot expect it to leave your work life intact. Try not to expect so much of yourself that you end up feeling overwhelmed and incapable. Remember that it is normal not to feel highly career-motivated when so much of your attention is on creating a family. One of the positive aspects of dealing with infertility is coming to understand what is really important to you. Facing up to career issues just might contribute to your life, helping you create a work situation that supports you in having a family.

Decisions about your career are complicated by the financial demands of infertility. Questions about work involve more than job satisfaction and salary: Should I find another position with a company that offers medical coverage? If I change jobs, could I end up losing maternity benefits just when I might need them? If I switch to part-time or quit, how will we afford the doctor's bills? The economic impact of infertility treatment can be just as disheartening as failing to conceive. As insurance companies continue to deny or cut back coverage for infertility claims, paying medical bills can be a real hardship even for fairly affluent couples.

But how can we put a price on having a child? It is difficult to "budget" what a child is worth to you; however, unless you face squarely the financial impact of pursuing pregnancy, you can find yourselves with a mountain of debt or living a life in which all your disposable income goes toward medical treatment. Some couples can take lifestyle restrictions longer than others can, but if treatment is not successful, at some point difficult choices have to be made.

Unfortunately, figuring out what you can afford to spend on having a baby is a part of learning to deal intelligently with an ever-increasing array of medical choices and decisions. Thanks to us belated baby-boomers, infertility research and treatment are also booming and becoming a multibillion-dollar-a-year business, and most of this money is paid for treatment that yields no results. This is not to say that treatment should not be pursued, only that unless you have substantial financial resources, you will need to make informed, rational decisions about your course of treatment—what, with whom, for how long, and at what cost.

The first decision, of course, is when to enter the maze. Some couples resist facing that their prefertile period is dragging on longer than they wanted or expected. While some people, like me, do not hesitate to run out and buy the basal thermometer and the *How to Get Pregnant* book, others resist even the smallest incursion of knowledge or technology into the process of creating life. They want it to happen "naturally." If you find yourself stuck in the early stages of the infertility maze, it may be because you don't want to acknowledge that it might take some unnatural acts to make something happen. The first act is to start educating yourself about your body and learning more than you ever wanted to know about the human reproductive process and how it goes awry. Several good books (listed in the bibliography) can help you learn the basics and teach you to track your cycle.

You will also need to decide when it's time to leave your good old gynecologist and seek out a fertility expert. Many gynecologists have very little training in infertility, technically known as "reproductive endocrinology." It requires at least two years of additional training, often including some experience with microsurgery and in vitro fertilization. Some doctors will tell you themselves when they have exhausted their expertise and will refer you to a specialist. Others may keep you hanging on longer than you want, figuring or hoping, as you are, that something will happen in time and perhaps not wanting to launch you unnecessarily into the expensive world of high-tech baby making. But some doctors may simply lack the skills and knowledge to diagnose a specific problem, and you may have to be the one to face up to that and decide to move on.

Finding a reproductive endocrinologist or fertility specialist is easier in large metropolitan areas; if you live elsewhere, you may need to travel. If there is a male problem, you will need to see a urologist or an andrologist who specializes in treating the male reproductive system. If your own doctor can't refer you to someone, or if you would like to contact several specialists, you can get a specialist reference list from the American Fertility Society or from RESOLVE (see "Resources, page 221).

If you have a choice of specialists, you may want to interview two or three to see whom you feel most comfortable with. Your fertility specialist will share your most intimate physical and emotional experiences, and it will help to have a good personal relationship as well as confidence in his or her professional abilities. Such can't always be the case, since some excellent, highly skilled doctors may lack a pleasing personality or the appropriate bedside manner, and choosing to work with one of these may mean you have to lower your expectations about the degree of emotional support you'll get. But even in the best of circumstances, the stress of treatment and your emotional strain can bring about miscommunication and misunderstandings. The best way to avoid them or resolve them quickly is to communicate openly and honestly, keeping in mind that you and your doctor are equal partners in the treatment process.

Keeping up your side of the partnership is crucial in the infertility labyrinth, where doctors seem to have the power of life or no life and the tendency is to turn yourselves over to them to "get fixed." It took some time for me to recognize doctors as the humans they are. It didn't happen until they started being the same age I was and I realized they couldn't be that much more sophisticated, especially having spent all that time in medical school while I was exploring the world and myself. (When one gynecologist I saw many years ago indicated he would like to do more than examine me during an exam, I ditched him, along with my last preconceptions about the medical priesthood.) Certainly, most doctors deserve our respect, but they don't deserve our reverence. They are not all-knowing authority figures whom you cannot question or get upset with. They also have enormous pressures from their work and cannot always give you the time and emotional support you need, even if they want to.

If you can't find a specialist you like, at least look for one who is willing to empower you with enough information to make sound, realistic decisions—someone who will work with you not so much as a patient but as a partner. Actually, you are not a patient in the traditional sense. You are not sick but seeking to get pregnant; and how that goal is achieved is a process of mutual decision making. Your doctor may suggest treatment you don't want. You may want to try procedures at a faster or slower rate. For you, participating as a partner means taking an active role, asking questions (even "stupid" ones) and letting the doctor know what you want and don't want. It is your responsibility to ask the questions and the doctor's (or his or her staff's) to answer them—in language and terms you can comprehend. Make sure you ask everything you want to know about procedures, timing, drugs and their side effects, and financial costs. If you are confused, ask for clarification. You may want to write the answers down so that you can be clear about what you heard and repeat it back. You may want to educate yourself further on your particular problem so you can interact knowledgeably. Don't hesitate to ask your doctor for printed material—books, articles, and journals you can read. Or contact sources such as RESOLVE to locate additional information.

If you do not receive the information and treatment you want from a doctor, or if you simply want to try someone else's expertise, remember that you have every right to get a second opinion and to switch doctors if you choose. I know this is sometimes difficult because of emotional bonds, unexpressed resentment, or fear that you will have to start all over again with someone you don't know. But changing doctors is not as hard as it seems. Simply inform your present doctor with a letter or a phone call that you would like to try another specialist and request that your records be sent there. Most doctors are quite comfortable with this procedure and will not take it personally. If you do want to offer personal criticism, or if you are upset or angry, it helps to communicate, even if only by letter. Try to be as clear and straightforward as possible about what displeases you. You might make some suggestions about how his or her practice could be improved, and let it go at that.

Probably the most important aspect of the doctor–patient relationship is having a joint game plan, a short- or long-term treatment strategy on which you agree. When we first saw Dr. B, he laid out a year's worth of treatment that he hoped would have us pregnant or at least knowing why not. He told us the costs of the tests, inseminations, and laparascopy and approximately what we would have to pay and when. As a year came around, we still had no pregnancy and no diagnosis, but we felt we at least had a completion of sorts. We had tried everything we had agreed to try, and we knew we had the choice of going ahead with adoption or trying more invasive, expensive fertility treatment.

Decisions about how far you will go, how much you will spend, and what you will endure physically and psychologically don't have to be made at the beginning of treatment. But it helps to know up front the range of choices available and to begin to consider the costs (both financial and emotional), the probabilities of success, and what issues need to be resolved in making your choices. Taking responsibility for your treatment means facing these realities and making decisions, not out of starry-eyed hope or blind determination, but with a clear vision of what you are willing and able to do to realize your dream of making a family.

Basically, the choices before a prefertile couple are: 1) to keep trying with no medical intervention; 2) to pursue various medical and surgical investigations to find and correct ovulation problems, pelvic problems, sperm problems (the "male factor"), or some combination of the three, or to treat habitual miscarriages; 3) to enter the brave new world of high-tech fertility treatment including in vitro fertilization (IVF) and gamete intrafallopian transfer (GIFT); 4) to bypass the male factor by having artificial insemination by donor (AID), a process with high success rates but sometimes complex emotional issues involved; 5) to try the risky business of finding a surrogate mother; 6) to adopt a child privately or through an agency; and 7) to decide to live without children.

Each of these seven options has costs and benefits, and each will have different meaning and value for different couples. With option 1, choosing not to do anything, you can still get pregnant, but it may take several years. You may save money but lose time, which may be okay if you are 25 but a real problem if you are over 35. Pursuing medical treatment, from mild interventions like taking Clomid to more invasive surgery, is a game of chance in which you are playing the odds. What are the chances that this drug or that procedure will get you pregnant? What are the costs in comparison to the likelihood of success? In order not to get stuck in the medical maze, you have to be realistic about your chances. To win, you have to conserve financial and emotional resources so that you can stay in the game. However expensive it gets, most couples find that they run out of emotional energy before they run out of money.

The initial investigatory process—the basic infertility work-up—usually follows the course that Bill and I took: *semen analysis* to determine sperm count and motility; *basal body temperature* readings to establish the length of the cycle and the probability of ovulation; *blood hormone level tests* in both men and women; *postcoital tests* to determine the interaction of the sperm and the cervical mucus; an *endometrial biopsy* to determine ovulation and hormone levels (one test I did not take); the *hysterosalpingogram* to examine the tubes and the uterus by X-ray; and the *laparoscopy* to inspect the tubes, uterus, and ovaries visually. In addition to these initial tests, your doctor may recommend other procedures such as checking for infections like chlamydia or examining the male for varicocele (dilated veins, like varicose veins) in the testicles.

After these various examinations, about 90 percent of infertility problems will be diagnosed. Generally, about 35 percent are attributed to female problems, 35 percent to male problems, and 20 percent to compound male and female problems. The remaining 10 percent are diagnosed as "infertility of unknown etiology," or unexplained infertility. Treatment for female problems includes drugs to enhance ovulation and surgery to clear up pelvic problems, such as endometriosis, blocked tubes, or uterine fibroid tumors, or to clear up problems around the cervix. Male infertility is more easily diagnosed but less easily treated. Usually, fertility drugs or surgery for varicocele will show results fairly quickly, whether they are successful or not. It's a good idea for the man to be checked out thoroughly early on before embarking on a female treatment program.

In pursuing medical investigations and surgical interventions, you can be as aggressive or as laid back as you want, providing, of course, you can find a doctor who is willing to move at your pace. Most physicians are scientists, predisposed to a slow, careful evaluation of problems and measured treatment, trying the least invasive and least expensive procedures first. That pace suits most patients early in the game, but as the years go by, couples become more and more impatient.

There are doctors who are willing to move directly and aggressively, but few prefertile couples really know what all their options are for speeding up diagnosis and treatment. And usually, if you want a more aggressive treatment process, you will have to push for it. That means educating yourself thoroughly about whatever you think your problem is, questioning your doctor about what he or she knows, and perhaps getting second and third opinions from other specialists. Don't let yourself get stuck in the maze for fear you'll hurt your doctor's feelings by pressing him or her or by investigating other approaches. Most doctors are very open to your input and to second opinions—or they should be.

Being completely informed and knowing what your chances are is particularly important if you are entering the most difficult part of the infertility maze—in vitro fertilization, or IVF, and gamete intrafallopian transfer, or GIFT. These two operations, you will recall, bring sperm and ripened eggs in direct contact: In IVF, they are combined in a laboratory dish where they fertilize to become embryos and are then transferred to the woman's uterus. This technique is recommended when the fallopian tubes are blocked or damaged. In GIFT, the egg and sperm mixture is placed directly in the fallopian tube, where fertilization can occur naturally. It requires at least one open tube and is usually recommended for couples who have sperm count problems or unexplained infertility. In both procedures, drugs such as Clomid, Pergonal, and recently Lupron are used to stimulate the production of eggs, and often as many as three to five eggs or four to six embryos are used. Both procedures can result in multiple births—usually twins, but also triplets and quadruplets. Another high-tech procedure, not nearly so common as IVF and GIFT, is embryo transfer: taking an embryo conceived in one body or in a laboratory dish and transferring it to another body. It may involve the use of donor eggs and sperm or even the use of a "host womb" if a woman is unable to carry a pregnancy.

The results of IVF and GIFT vary according to the woman's age and the presence of a male factor. Although the technology of all these procedures is developing rapidly, the results being achieved now, in the late 1980s, are still disappointing given the high costs and the physical and emotional demands on a couple. GIFT seems to offer the greatest promise, with live birth success rates ranging between 15 and 30 percent and costs running between $3000 and $6000. IVF still has not passed the 20 percent live birth bench mark (usually 10 percent), although costs continue to climb—now up to $8000 in some programs.

Deciding to pursue these treatments may not be an entirely rational decision. Probably, it won't be. Hope springs eternal in the hearts of the prefertile, and some who have been trying everything for so long may see the success rates as a glass one-fifth full rather than four-fifths empty. And, of course, no one can tell you what is right for you. What seems like an ill-advised obsession may be considered great determination and perseverance if it works. Trying to find the fine line between blind obsession and clear-sighted perseverance, I think of Michele and Wendy, two women who have spent an inordinate amount of time, energy, and money on their fertility treatment.

Michele was 45 years old when a mutual friend introduced us. She and her husband Alan, who was 47, were both psychotherapists, and they had been Trying since they got married three years earlier. Michele had been pregnant at age 20 and had had a late-term abortion that left her cervical tissue severely damaged. At the time, it didn't quite sink in when the doctor told her, "You know, now you'll never be able to have children." She took birth control pills anyway during her twenties but stopped in her late thirties to see if she could get pregnant. She wasn't really concerned about her age as a factor in infertility, assuming she could conceive until menopause in her fifties. Early in their relationship, when they were living together, Alan wasn't interested in babies, having raised two adopted children in his first marriage. But once they were married, they decided to go for it, and Michele began her odyssey through the maze. She had seen three specialists before she finally had surgery to improve her cervical opening. Then she began intrauterine insemination.

She, too, saw Dr. B, and had prevailed upon him to do fifteen inseminations—nine more than he would normally do. She'd been on high doses of Clomid for two years and felt severe emotional side effects—fragility and irrationality similar to what people associate with premenstrual syndrome. (One woman referred to it as "the Bambi–Hitler syndrome.") At the same time, she was seeing an acupuncturist twice a week and taking herbs. In two years, she and Alan spent over $20,000 on these various treatments.

A year later, when I contacted Michele again to see how things were going, she had been to two more specialists and had spent another $10,000 on inseminations with Pergonal. She was considering doing the GIFT procedure, although her only open tube had some adhesions. We met to talk at a trendy Berkeley cafe, and during our conversation a young mother with a small baby had the bad taste to occupy the table next to us. Tears streamed down Michele's cheeks as she recounted the familiar litany of the infertile. She felt her life was on hold, that she couldn't make plans, that she could only live day to day. She and Alan had been through a lot of bad times in their relationship, but now she felt it was stronger than ever, even though their sexual energy was practically nil. She knew that Alan would be thrilled if she could resolve not to have children, but she just couldn't face being "childfree," a euphemism she hated. "It's like a woman whose husband has left her after twenty years exclaiming that she's 'husband-free'."

Both Michele and Alan felt scared and ambivalent about adoption—Alan more so than she—and she felt the only reason he was still going along with the treatment was that if it worked, he wouldn't have to deal with adopting. Having found complete fulfillment in adoption, I wanted to encourage Michele in that direction, but it was clear she planned to continue her quest to the end, whether bitter or sweet. At 46, she would soon be at the age at which specialists would decline to work with her, so there was one wave of last-ditch fertility effort before she would consider adoption. Was this woman ridiculously obsessed or incredibly brave and courageous?

Most people who knew Wendy, also a psychotherapist who lives in Berkeley, asked the same question about her. I had known Wendy back in the early seventies, when she and her psychologist husband, Nathan, were at the center of a big group of politically active, socially conscious friends. Blessed with family money, Wendy and Nathan had a huge house in the Berkeley hills and a farm in the country, and they envisioned a large family to inhabit them. They had a son and then adopted a daughter, but they suspended having more children while Wendy went back to graduate school. She used a Dalkon Shield for birth control, never suspecting that the cramps and infections she was experiencing were linked to that deadly device. It was removed in 1973, but it wasn't until after a couple of years of mystery over why she wasn't getting pregnant that a hysterosalpingogram revealed that both tubes were closed. She had two laparotomies to clear the tubes and was about to have another when she heard about in vitro fertilization.

She and Nathan went directly to the source, the clinic in Bourn, England (a nicely named location), where Louise Brown had become the first baby conceived in a petri dish.

Wendy and Nathan's first in vitro attempt took place at Bourn in 1982, and over the next four years, they traveled to four other locations and had eight complete in vitro procedures. If you counted all the times Wendy took Pergonal that were not consummated in the operation for one reason or another, the number of attempts would be around twice that many. After one procedure, she was told she was pregnant, only to find a day or so later that she'd gotten someone else's blood test results. When she was 39, after more than ten years and over $100,000 worth of treatment, Wendy got pregnant on in vitro number eight, and baby Christopher came along at last.

Of course, having money, some insurance coverage, and a settlement from the Dalkon Shield people contributed to Wendy's financial resources, but the physical and emotional energy involved in her long trip through the labyrinth is truly astonishing. She knew that she might never get pregnant, that she was going to have to put out an enormous amount of effort for possibly no results, but she kept at it. "Technology made me infertile," she said, "and I was determined that it would make me fertile again." She was encouraged by a woman she'd met in Bourn who'd gotten pregnant on her seventh try, and she carried a letter from her in her purse.

Each attempt was going to be the last one, and she began to worry she'd never stop—"the world's first IVF junkie." Friends said, "Oh no, I thought you weren't going to do that again, you must be crazy," and she stopped telling her mother about it because she was worried Wendy was being "experimented on." But Nathan supported her. "There's no reason this shouldn't work sometime," he said and left it up to her. Wendy attributes her success to the ancient Chinese saying "Perseverance furthers," and to her own self-education. She became a lay expert on the in vitro process, learning everything she could, studying medical papers and research, and working closely with her last doctor to pin down the precise factors that would make it work. Her last three attempts were with a doctor in Berkeley who had given her a great deal of close personal attention (unlike other IVF "factories" she'd been through). His ability to play around with the various factors —dosage of Pergonal, blood hormone levels, and so forth— was what paid off. It was not, as Wendy emphasized, "magical thinking" or "relaxing" that had anything to do with it. It was "scientific knowledge gleaned and acted upon" plus dogged determination.

For every Wendy, however, there are eight or nine determined souls who get nothing but heartbreak out of in vitro. In seeking out an in vitro program, couples try to find one with a high success rate, but the percentages of success reported by various clinics may be based on different criteria. Some may indicate the pregnancy rate only of the women who have had eggs transferred. Some may include all pregnancies reported without correcting for ectopic pregnancies and miscarriages. The best indicator of a true success rate is the number of live births in relation to the number of women who started the program. Success rates go up according to the number of embryos transferred, but so do the chances of multiple births.

When an IVF attempt fails, the impact is especially devastating. Having an embryo transferred often makes a woman feel pregnant, and when she learns she is not, there is a true sense of loss, just as there is with an early miscarriage. It's not surprising that few women can match Wendy's perseverance. Playing the IVF odds is usually a difficult, painful game, and—face it—there are few lucky winners.

While the odds with GIFT are somewhat better and the process a little less expensive and invasive, the emotional risks are the same. I have great respect for the courage of couples who go this route, and great compassion for those who try once or twice and give up. Perseverance furthers ... sometimes.

Some people feel a half-biological baby is better than none

and decide to use someone else's sperm or eggs. Donor eggs are now being used in IVF and GIFT programs for women who cannot produce enough of their own. Often, women want the eggs to be provided by someone close to them—a sister, cousin, or friend—but sometimes they come from anonymous donors. More common, however, is the use of donor sperm for Artificial Insemination by Donor, or AID. If the problem is male sperm, AID is a fairly simple, inexpensive solution. Sperm donors (usually medical students) are carefully screened for any medical problems or infections, and couples can choose a donor on the basis of coloring, height, and other characteristics, including religion. The insemination is done by a doctor, and success rates are high—40 to 80 percent within six months. In recent years, the AIDS epidemic has led to the use of frozen sperm, kept for three to six months while the donor is tested for HIV, the AIDS virus. However, results with frozen sperm are somewhat lower.

But while the process of donor insemination is simple, choosing the method is often complex. Deciding on AID as a pregnancy option means you must consider and resolve the psychological and emotional issues of involving a third, usually anonymous, person in making your baby. Many infertile couples get stuck at this juncture in the maze—only about 5 percent of couples with a male factor problem pursue this option. Most commonly, the objection to the process comes from the husband, who finds he can't accept the idea of his wife's being impregnated by another man or feels he can't accept "another man's child." Both husband and wife may be put off by the possible legal and social issues, so it's a good idea to be thoroughly informed about the laws regarding AID paternity in your state.

Deciding on AID can involve many of the same issues in deciding to adopt, although you have a far greater degree of control. Generally, you will know more about the biological father than you will in an adoption, and you can ensure good prenatal care and nutrition during the pregnancy. But there are still the same questions: "Should we just keep it a secret from everyone?" "What and how do we tell our child about his or her biological father?" "Will he or she want to know or find him?" Getting comfortable with AID means examining many basic attitudes and your readiness to let go of a "normal" biological birth. It's a decision on which couples must align, both husband and wife feeling completely open to a process that will continue for many years after birth.

Jonathan and Penny decided to try AID after cancer of the testicles made it impossible for Jonathan to produce effective sperm. Penny at first pushed for adoption, afraid that Jonathan would be uncomfortable with her "being pregnant by another man." Even though she very much wanted to experience pregnancy and childbirth, she didn't push for AID. When it came up in their RESOLVE support group discussions, Jonathan was able to share some of his fears and soon started feeling more positive about having a baby that would be "at least half ours." Penny was pregnant after their first insemination, and then it really struck them. Their immediate family and close friends knew about the circumstances of the pregnancy, but what would they tell other relatives and acquaintances? What would they tell their child?

When baby Larry was born, any lingering doubts about their decision were dispelled by their baby's first cry. As they fell head over heels in love with their beautiful red-haired boy, his actual paternity seemed completely irrelevant—even more so as he seemed to grow into "the spitting image of his father." After much soul searching, Jonathan and Penny decided to be open about the situation should questions arise, but they didn't go around volunteering the information. For the most part, people who knew reacted thoughtfully and tactfully. Only an annoying aunt and uncle found it necessary to publicly pronounce at every family gathering "how much Larry looks like both of you. You'd never guess he had another father...."

On these and other occasions, Jonathan and Penny found themselves admitting that they sometimes wished they could have just kept the whole thing a secret. "Who really needs to know?" They are still contemplating what and how they will tell little Larry.

Couples who do embrace having a child with the help of donor sperm are often amazed that the practice isn't more common. For some there may be religious or ethical objections (it is forbidden by the Roman Catholic Church and by Orthodox Judaism), but many couples can find their questions answered and their fears assuaged by good counseling. The decision may be a complex and difficult one, but AID may be the fastest, easiest route to what you want—a family.

Surrogate motherhood is a far riskier way of having a half-biological child. An anonymous sperm donor who ejaculates into a jar obviously plays a very different role than a woman who carries a child for nine months just beneath her heart. But how does she differ from the woman who decides to give up her baby for adoption? Why the legal furor over surrogacy to the point of banning it in some states while adoption remains legal throughout the country?

Although surrogacy has been practiced since Biblical days when Sarah's maid Hagar bore a child, Ishmael, for Abraham, there has been little or no regulation of the process. Surrogacy as an alternative for infertile couples has gained recognition only in the past ten years as surrogate parenting clinics have been established. It gained public notoriety when surrogate mother Mary Beth Whitehead refused to give up the child she had borne and went to court in an effort to retain custody. Eventually, the father and his wife won custody and legally adopted Baby M, but Mary Beth Whitehead retains extensive visitation rights.

The Whitehead case resolved little in the surrogacy furor, leaving open the question of whether surrogate parenting contracts are legal. The fundamental difference from adoption, of course, is that the surrogate mother is paid a sum of money—the going rate is $10,000—for her "services" as an egg donor and womb. (The couple may pay up to $20,000 more in clinic and legal expenses.)

The commercialization of childbearing raises profound legal and ethical issues for society and for individuals contemplating surrogacy. As a society, we have to face the implications of poor women bearing children for rich couples, of relegating motherhood to a contractual proposition, and of trying to enforce a contract by taking a child from its mother. Couples contemplating contract motherhood (perhaps a more accurate term for surrogacy) must delve deeply into their attitudes and emotions before embarking on such a risky route to parenthood: Can you afford the $20,000 to $30,000 the process costs? Do you both equally desire the surrogacy solution? (As men can feel "left out" of AID, surrogacy can make women feel estranged, inadequate, and even sexually jealous.) Do you feel comfortable with the ethical issues of paying a woman to carry your child? What sort of relationship do you want with the contract mother—how well do you want to get to know her? How involved will you be medically in her pregnancy (such as requiring amniocentesis or other screening)? What will you do if a problem is detected or there is a miscarriage? How will you proceed if the birth mother changes her mind and wants to keep the baby? Are you prepared to experience the pain and guilt that may result from an unhappy experience on the part of the birth mother? What and how will you tell your child about the circumstances of his or her birth?

Many professionals in the surrogacy field as well as surrogates and parents say that the issue has been blown out of proportion. They say that, for most people, the surrogate or contract mother arrangement works perfectly well, leaving all parties happy and satisfied. There are those unique women who enjoy being pregnant, who genuinely want to give the gift of life to an infertile couple, and who are able to disengage themselves emotionally from their child and his or her family. Some even refuse to accept money other than what will cover direct costs. Others who do take money see it not as an obligation, but as "an exchange of gifts."

Aaron, 48, and Pat, 43, were planning to adopt when a friend of a friend offered to become a surrogate mother for them. Divorced and the mother of a 10-year-old boy, Linda loved being pregnant and the idea of helping a couple have a family. At first, Pat was reluctant because of all the legal hassles, but Aaron was thrilled. Most of his family had died in the Holocaust, and he felt blessed to have an opportunity to continue his family's genealogy. They met Linda, liked her immediately, and were convinced by her excitement and sincerity. Aaron and Pat had decided beforehand that if Linda changed her mind at any point, they would not fight it legally. To avoid any problems, they structured their agreement as a "prearranged adoption." The insemination was carried out by a licensed doctor, and Aaron had no paternity claims—he was simply a sperm donor. There would be no payment for services; rather, Linda would receive the normal support payments that are legal under the state's adoption laws as well as payment of all medical and legal fees. When they found out the first insemination "took," Aaron, Pat, and Linda celebrated together and have continued to remain in close communication throughout the pregnancy. Linda and her son received some counseling during the process, and as they await the birth, all parties have only the most positive feelings.

Other couples I know who have had children borne by surrogate mothers also report a positive experience on all sides. We hear little in the media about these cases, as most people prefer to keep their arrangement a private matter. But we also do not hear much from those women, less assertive than Mary Beth Whitehead, for whom having given up a child continues to be emotionally distressing. As with adoption, there is a range of opinion and practice regarding contact between the couple and the birth mother. Some clinics prefer anonymity, but there seems to be a trend toward encouraging contact. Personal relationships allow for building mutual caring and trust, both of which are at the heart of the surrogate parenting process.

The future of surrogate or contract parenting is a hazy one. In the past decade, only about 1000 babies have been born through such contracts, but surrogacy clinics expect to be serving 1000 to 2000 couples a year soon—unless, of course, legal limitations are established. Michigan has recently joined five other states in making it a felony to establish a parenting contract; other states are struggling with the issue. I find myself feeling as ambivalent as many legislators must feel—aware of the potential for the exploitation of women and yet recognizing the feelings that lead both infertile couples and birth mothers into participating. Recently, I thought about the biblical story of Sarah and Hagar and realized I couldn't remember how it turned out. I found a Bible and read that, on Sarah's demand, Abraham banished both Hagar and Ishmael into the desert. Apparently, it was as risky then as it is now.

Almost every unconventional method of having a child, from IVF to AID to surrogacy, involves certain ethical and moral issues. For some people these are easily resolved, but for others they pose serious questions about basic beliefs. Is AID a form of adultery? Is it morally wrong, as the Catholic Church says, for sperm and egg to be brought together in a glass dish rather than in the process of human intercourse? What rights does an embryo have? Is it a human life or is it property to be dealt with or disposed of by doctors? Is it morally right for a host womb mother to carry another couple's child? Will contract motherhood lead to an epidemic of poor women bearing rich couples' babies?

Whatever route you follow toward creating your family, you will need to give thought to the ethics inherent in any type of "unnatural" parenting, even adoption. Whether or not you have religious beliefs, the questions raised are yours to grapple with and yours to answer—for yourselves, not for anyone else in the world. If you are bothered by moral concerns, seek help, perhaps from more than one perspective, and give yourself the time to feel certain that the course you embark upon is right for you.

If one of the options covered here brings you a child, you won't have to face the agonizing decision of when to end your journey through the infertility labyrinth. Knowing when to stop is one of the most difficult decisions couples have to face, for there are always new technologies and new doctors who may yet lead you out of the maze. But if the quest begins to take on a quixotic feeling, if your emotions and finances just can't bear any more stretching, perhaps you are ready for a new adventure.

What's at the end of the infertility maze? Couples who have run the gamut of infertility treatment options without results face the final choice of adopting or living without children. Before looking deeper into the issues surrounding adoption in the next chapter, it is important to acknowledge the honesty and courage of couples who choose to be "childfree." The word itself has come into use as an alternative to the term "childless," which implies that something is missing. Certainly, what is missed by not having children can be made up for in many ways—by having special relationships with other people's children, including foster children, by pursuing career interests or working for causes, by having the time, money, and freedom to travel or develop hobbies and avocations, and by having the opportunity to focus on the marriage relationship, nurturing and deepening it. The prejudice against families of two—the notion that they are selfish or inadequate or destined for a lonely old age—is waning as it becomes apparent that most "dinks" (double income, no kids) are having a great time in life, enjoying themselves and finding fulfillment in their work and in all kinds of relationships.

Choosing this lifestyle after years of waiting and working for a baby can be a momentous decision. It works out best if it is indeed a definite decision and not a slow slide into "no man's land," that is, not doing anything about it but still hoping it happens and still feeling the pain and disappointment. Not to decide is to decide. Some couples find it useful after making their decision to start using birth control again to help clarify their position. Of course, it also helps if both partners are equally resolved. Supporting each other in making the choice and in creating new life goals together can be a powerful and inspiring experience for a couple—not the same as having a child but just as strengthening and life affirming.

I believe it is important to give serious thought to what your life could be like without children and to open up to this possibility. You may find it to be more appealing than you imagined. At the very least, giving it consideration will help you clarify your feelings about adoption. If you do choose the childfree path, God Bless. If you believe you can't be happy without children, read on.

Chapter Eight

Successful Adoption

*L*ike the infertility odyssey, the adoption process can also seem like a maze of unexpected hurdles, dead ends, and frustrating failures. There just aren't any babies out there, we are told, and the wait for an infant is years long. It seems the only adoption stories we hear about in the media are the ones where things went wrong: the father turns out to be a child abuser; the teenage mother returns to claim her baby and devastates a couple's life; a young woman and her boyfriend are arrested for trying to "sell" her baby to a number of desperate couples. The conventional wisdom about adoption today is not only that it is dangerous, but that it is so difficult that few couples can expect to find a healthy newborn of the color they choose.

It is true that the adoption situation in this country has changed radically since the late sixties, when agencies had a plentiful supply of unwed mothers who had no alternative but to give up their babies. This was before the days of widely available contraceptives and legal abortions and a cultural light-year away from general public acceptance of single mothers raising babies on their own (albeit usually with the assistance of public welfare). Girls with protruding bellies walking high school halls are no longer a source of scandal and shame, and some schools have so many pregnant girls that they have their own special classes together (giving new meaning to the term "alma mater"). Now, in the eighties, there is more sex, more pregnancy, more contraception, and more abortion, and fewer babies available for adoption. Today, it is estimated that 70 to 90 percent of all single women who bear babies keep them.

As the adoption supply side has been shrinking, the demand side has been growing, filling up with those of us who delayed childbearing, who suffer unexplained or untreatable infertility, or who can't tolerate financially or psychically the fertility treatment grind. In response to the glut of would-be adopters, adoption agencies now find children only for those couples considered "most desirable"—young (usually under 35), healthy (no handicaps), well-educated, financially stable, not previously married, with a "strong" traditional relationship (preferably a wife who does not have a demanding career), and flexibility with regard to the type of child they will accept. If you fit this description, you get to join a waiting list five years long.

Fortunately, this is not the entire story. In fact, it is estimated that less than half of today's adoptions take place through traditional agencies. Couples who want to adopt are seeking out babies independently—and finding them through private adoption. Thousands of birth mothers are choosing the private adoption route, and more will do so as they come to know about it. The growing phenomenon of private or independent adoption provides an important new avenue for adoptive couples who do not fit the agency mold, as well as for single people. It has made it possible for me to say that if you decide to adopt, no matter how old you are or what your circumstances are, and you do the work involved, you can have one, two, or more babies to create the family you want.

Knowing that babies are available may be all some couples need to get going, but more likely there is first the difficult process of deciding to adopt. For some, the choice before them is quite clear. They are truly infertile, have tried all the remedies, and know adoption is the only path to a family. For others, unexplained infertility and access to ever more treatment opportunities means there is always the hope of a "miracle child." They either have to let go of their fantasy or pursue both routes at the same time—a highly demanding, potentially exhausting experience. In either case, making the choice to pursue adoption means shifting your focus from getting pregnant to getting a baby.

Getting a baby requires a lot of energy and effort, so it is best to have made a clear decision that, more than anything, you want to be a parent. That may not be the case for everyone. Although friends and family may assume adoption is the obvious solution to infertility, wanting to give birth to your own baby is not the same as wanting any baby. Just because you cannot have a child of your own does not mean you are obligated to adopt. Feeling pressured into adopting could affect how you feel about your adopted child or cause problems in your family relationships. It is important to realize that choosing not to adopt is not a decision to feel guilty or defensive about. It may bring new clarity to your life and enable you to pursue other options.

If you do feel you want parenthood above all else, make sure that the decision is a mutual one. Often, couples do not share the same feelings about adoption. The disparity may be small and easy to work out, or it may be a major crisis of relationship requiring much soul searching, discussion, and counseling over time. Even if both partners are ready at the same time, past years of discouragement may make it difficult to feel

excited and enthusiastic about what lies ahead. It may not be
necessary for both partners to feel absolutely thrilled about
adopting, but there must at least be a general good feeling
about it, even though some doubts and misgivings may continue. Remember that people who get pregnant don't always
feel great about what they are doing either.

Feeling okay about moving on to a new focus is at the heart
of resolving your infertility. To be ready to receive, it seems, you
have to be ready to let go. You need to be willing to give up your
attachment to your unborn child, though you may certainly still
hope for his or her appearance. Much is made these days, especially in adoption agencies, of the need to resolve your infertility before you decide to adopt. I'm not sure that's possible.
Letting go is a process that happens over time. I doubt that any
of us feel completely resolved about letting go of the dream of
"our own" baby before we hold a baby in our arms who we
know is "our" baby even though he or she came from another.
Even with Alexander in our lives, this perfect child whom I adore
completely, I would still like another baby that "we made."

Resolving your infertility does not mean not wanting to
get pregnant anymore or no longer feeling sad or resentful
about what you have gone through. It does mean healing your
self-esteem and self-worth and letting go of feelings of failure
and inadequacy. It means believing that you and your spouse,
like any other good people, have a right to raise a child—even
a completely healthy child or maybe two healthy children—
and having confidence that you can and will do so joyously.
The healing that needs to go on around your infertility may
take time, and it may go on while you are raising an adopted
child. Adoption does not in itself resolve infertility (or cure
it, as everyone would have you believe), but it does give you
what you want: a child to love.

The first fear to surface when you think about adopting
is whether you will indeed love that child fully, completely,
or even enough. It is so hard to imagine that the offspring of

two strangers could find a place in your heart comparable to the one you reserved for "our child." Though it is empty, it is a holy place, reserved for someone of your own flesh and blood—not some unknown quantity. How can you know you will love what you don't know?

I remember, when we were thinking about adopting, going about the world scrutinizing every child I saw. What if that were my baby? Could I possibly love that boy with the ears sticking out or the little girl throwing a tantrum in the super-market aisle? My friends kept reminding me that there were no sure things with biological children—they, too, had weird features and behaved like brats. These comments didn't really convince me, so I just had to make a leap of faith. I had to trust my own capacity to love and my own maternal instincts, and I had to trust Bill, who never had any doubt about loving a child that was not our own. Now, I smile inside when people who are thinking about adopting ask me about loving or "bond-ing with" a child. I wish I could give them scientific evidence or the results of some survey, but I can only say, I'm sorry, the only evidence I have is my experience—and that of every adoptive couple I have talked to: The instant you lay eyes on that baby, you will be madly in love. Of course, whether they are adopted or not, difficult babies can cause a real strain on new parents. Adoptive parents may feel particularly sensitive about any negative feelings, but over time they develop the same attachment as any other parents.

If you are able to make that leap of faith and feel you can love someone else's baby, you may then find yourself facing all the embarrassing questions you are afraid to admit you have: Will he or she be beautiful? intelligent? good-humored? of good physique? You are supposed to care only about the child's health. Don't all expectant parents say, "We'll just be happy if the baby's healthy," even though they may be dying for a girl or a boy? You feel you should not be concerned about the color of his hair or whether she will have what it takes to get into Harvard. You are particularly not supposed to be concerned about whether he or she will look like you, and you should consider yourselves lucky if you can find a child with all limbs and faculties intact.

However petty your concerns may seem, it is vital that you let them come to the surface and examine them. You need to talk about them, especially with your partner and perhaps with friends, a therapist, or an adoption counselor. You may not resolve them completely, but at least you will be aware of your fears, fantasies, and ambivalences. Keep in mind that "natural" parents have the same concerns about their babies and may be just as ambivalent about having them, yet nobody has to certify that it's okay for them to have a child.

There are other very real issues to be considered, such as what you will do if there is something wrong with the baby. Are you obliged to take a child born with mental or physical defects? Will you want to? These are questions often asked but seldom faced in reality. Nevertheless, if the baby you have been waiting for (and paying for) does turn out to have serious problems, you need to be prepared or at least have access to expert advice. In private adoption, you are not obligated to take a child until after you have signed the adoption papers, so you need to know about the baby's health before you do so. Your lawyer or adoption counselor should be able to advise you on this matter.

Another question is how your families will react. Will the baby be treated like all the other nephews, nieces, and cousins? Will Grandma be secretly heartbroken or Grandpa nervous about relating to "someone else's child"? Don't just wonder about it; talk to the people in your family who you know will be affected. We were surprised to find our families so enthusiatic about our moving on adoption. You may find, as we did, that they are less hung up about it than you are.

Often, fears and concerns about adoption are not so much about the baby or others but about yourselves. Isn't this just another impossible dream to pursue? Are we up to facing what may be another long string of disappointments? What if we never find a baby? What if we do get a baby right away—are we really ready to be parents? What would we do if the mother changed her mind and wanted the baby back? How could we face such a loss? The questions are all valid and need to be examined at some point in the process. But don't get paralyzed by "what ifs" before you even begin. The most important part of deciding to adopt is having a positive, optimistic attitude, knowing there is a baby out there for you and being willing to press through all barriers to find it.

Once you have determined that you want to adopt, you will need to familiarize yourselves with your options: going through an agency or pursuing private adoption. If you are young, not in a desperate hurry, or perhaps still undergoing fertility treatment, you may choose the agency route knowing that you may have to wait a few years for an infant. You may also go to an agency if you are interested in an older child or a child with special problems. If you are over 35 or want a newborn baby within a year, however, private adoption is the only way to go.

There are many benefits to adopting through the agency system—it is usually less expensive and may require less personal involvement than private adoption. Adoptive parents can be assured of medical screening of the child and appropriate legal relinquishment, and they may sometimes receive counseling. But these advantages are meaningless if you simply aren't acceptable or accepted.

I never made it past the first phone call to a local adoption agency—there was a dead silence when I told them I was 41— nor do I know anyone who has adopted through an agency in the past five years. So, I cannot speak with experience about pursuing an agency adoption, although it is obviously a workable alternative for some people. Before you start contacting agencies, I highly recommend that you read *Beating the Adoption Game* by Cynthia D. Martin. This excellent book tells you what you need to know about dealing with adoption agencies as well as about how to pursue other alternatives, such as foreign adoption, adoption of special needs children, and private adoption.

Despite warnings from the agency establishment that it is dangerous and possibly illegal, 50 to 80 percent of infants are placed independently without any agency involvement (in California, 90 percent of adoptions are private). Private or independent adoption actually refers to the placement of the baby through nonagency contacts. Once the baby is placed, the process follows the same route as agency adoptions and involves whatever state agency is responsible, usually the social services/public welfare department. Private adoption is legal in all but six states. It is distinguished from black market adoption, or baby selling, in that any exchange of money follows the state's legal guidelines—that is, certain payments are legal (pregnancy and birth medical expenses, some basic living costs) and others are not. Reputable attorneys or adoption counselors can help ensure that the process is legal, but problems can arise over what expenses are appropriate. Some adoptions may thus end up in the "gray market" category, although most do not.

Private adoption means that adoptive parents must locate a child themselves, usually through personal contacts, through a mass mailing to professionals who come in contact with pregnant women, or, in some states, through classified ads in the newspaper. Some lucky people may, as Bill and I did, stumble into a ready-made adoption situation. Even though there are few storks out there like Scott Roberts, I know of several couples outside the Oklahoma connection who found babies quickly and easily. A friend of ours who owns a travel agency had had three miscarriages, and a client who knew about it called her about a young birth mother even before our friend and her husband had decided to adopt. They had a baby boy within a few days. Another couple sent out 100 letters and received a call immediately. They were parents within two weeks. These stories are the exceptions, but most couples I know have found their babies within a year of beginning their search. One couple did not hear anything for almost two years, but the only call that came brought them their baby girl in just a few days.

The first place to begin is with your friends and families and the people they know. Most people, by the way, don't really know much about private adoption, and you will need to educate folks about the process so they can help you. Chances are they've felt helpless for so long, it will be great for them to finally be able to do something for you by providing people to contact. You just have to keep in mind the old saying, "You are never more than three people away from anyone in the world." Someone you contact will have contact with someone who will have contact with a pregnant woman who wants to give up her child. It is estimated that there will be a million to a million and a half pregnant teenagers in the next year, as well as tens of thousands of older women who will have unwanted pregnancies. One of them could bear a child that will become yours.

Cynthia Martin's *Beating the Adoption Game* will tell you all you need to know about creating a strategy for finding your child. While a mass mailing to gynecologists and high school counselors can work, adoption lawyers and counselors will all tell you that personal contacts will yield the greatest success. One woman I know got in touch with her college alumni director and was able to get the names and addresses of her classmates who were in the medical profession. She sent personal letters to each of them—about 100 people—and received 20 replies indicating support. Although she ended up getting her baby through another contact, she is ready to write her classmates again about a second child. Another couple I know gave out letters to their friends' teenage daughters and asked them to pass them around their high schools. Within a few weeks, a young girl, six months pregnant, contacted them, and three months later they were parents. Friends of mine, Jane and Peter, advertised in a newspaper in Oregon: "Loving, financially secure California couple seeks to adopt infant into happy home. Legal and medical expenses covered. Oregon attorney involved. Call Jane or Peter collect...." The ad ran for a couple of weeks, and one Sunday they received a call from a birth grandmother inviting them to come up and meet her daughter, who had just given birth the night before. Three days later, baby Victoria came home with them.

The bottom line on finding a baby is patience, perserverance, and creativity. Says Cynthia Martin: "*You* are the only limit on the number of possible contacts. Children are available for adoption if you search long enough and thoroughly enough.... Above all, in a baby search you must be bold. Believing that there is a child out there for you, you must be willing to venture forth to find him or her. Timidity will leave you childless. The people who find a child are those who boldly go after one."

Being optimistic about finding a child does not mean ignoring the potential problems and risks—it means knowing what difficulties could arise and being prepared to deal with them. There are fraudulent situations and unscrupulous people out there. Recently in California, a young woman promised her unborn child to several couples and absconded with tens of thousands of dollars paid for "living expenses." It turned out the girl was not even pregnant. A couple we know traveled to Hawaii to meet a birth mother who promised them her baby, but two days before it was born, the birth grandmother called demanding a cashiers check for $10,000. When they referred her to their lawyer, they got word the girl had changed her mind and was keeping the baby.

You may be lucky if you find out your adoption isn't going to work out before you actually get the baby. In private adoption situations, the birth mother may change her mind and reclaim the baby at any time before she signs the consent to adoption papers. Having a baby taken back by a birth mother after you have cared for and bonded with him or her is every adoptive parent's worst nightmare, and for some it is a life-shattering reality. It is one of the reasons people find private adoption so dangerous. You may have to wait years for an agency adoption, but when you get the child (usually several weeks or a few months after birth) you know he or she cannot be taken away.

There is no way to minimize the heartbreak of losing a baby you believed to be yours, one you have loved and changed and nursed and rocked and showed off to friends and family. This happened to two couples I know: Joanne and Lyle had their baby for a few days; Elaine and Joe had theirs for several weeks. Both were private, open adoptions in which the couples knew the birth mothers and had significant contact with them before the births. When the birth mothers changed their minds, both couples were devastated, feeling as desolate as any parents whose infant had just died. Joanne and Lyle immediately began searching for another baby, and when two birth mothers contacted them at about the same time, they decided to take both babies. They now have a daughter and a son a month apart in age.

Having lived with their baby longer, Elaine and Joe felt completely drained emotionally by their loss and stayed depressed for many months. Afraid of another disappointment, they could not find the strength to pursue adoption again. Beverly, my friend who had referred us to Scott Roberts, was acquainted with Elaine, who worked for her gynecologist. She knew about Elaine and Joe's ordeal and felt deeply for them but had never talked to Elaine about it. One day when Beverly was driving past her doctor's office, she had a strange experience. "It was as if a mysterious force just took over and drove me into the parking lot," she said. "Even though I barely knew Elaine, I knew that I wanted to refer her to Scott Roberts." Joe and Elaine were suspicious and even a bit paranoid, but within a few months Scott arranged the adoption of their son, Jay. Their utter ecstasy at being parents of a beautiful baby has assuaged some of their sadness, but the loss has left its scars. They waited five months to send out Jay's birth announcement.

There is no way to guarantee you won't have problems with an adoption, but the risks are in no way as great as the potential reward. You need not expect the worst, but you can be prepared for it by being as careful as possible in arranging your adoption. It may help to have the advice of a lawyer or adoption counselor you trust. There are a growing number of attorneys whose primary business is arranging adoptions, and recently a number of lay counselors and private agencies have entered the field—generally people who themselves have adopted and want to make adoption more available to other couples. While they do not find the birth mother for you, they serve as liaisons and counselors for both birth parents and adoptive couples and are available to help mediate should any problems arise.

However you go about your private adoption search, it is important to see yourself not as a passive recipient but as an active agent, able to take responsibility for and shape what is happening. How you behave in a difficult situation with a birth mother can make a big difference and possibly save an adoption. Keep in mind that with adoption, as opposed to fertility treatment, the odds are with you. According to Cynthia Martin, only about 12 percent of private adoptions get into trouble, and half of those are resolved when all parties listen and respond to each other's needs. Another quarter are resolved with hard work, so that only 3 percent of all private adoptions are "aborted." Others in the adoption field bear out these statistics—only 3 to 5 percent of babies placed are reclaimed (although no one knows how many birth mothers change their minds up to and during birth). Generally, a failed adoption, though painful, provides the experience needed to make the next try a success.

If you have decided to go after a child, and if you live in an area where open adoption is popular (the West Coast now but heading East), you may want to begin thinking about the issues posed by having contact with a birth mother or birth parents. Probably, your first tendency will be, as ours was, to reject the idea as frightening and hope and pray that the birth mother you find will want no contact with you. But in today's adoption world, even if you go through an agency, you may need to consider your relationship with the birth parents and make some decisions about it.

It is important that you recognize that the term "open adoption" covers a very wide range of options. The spectrum goes something like this: Scenario 1: The birth parent(s) choose(s) the adoptive parents, and they know about each other. Scenario 2: Birth parent(s) and adoptive parents meet each other in person a few times before the birth and then exchange letters and pictures after the baby is born. Scenario 3: The birth mother comes to live with the adoptive couple during her pregnancy, and they attend the birth as labor coaches; afterwards, the birth mother visits the child occasionally at agreed-on times. Scenario 4: The birth parent(s) and adoptive parents maintain a close, familial relationship with regular visits much like close relatives have.

Scenario 4, at the farthest end of the spectrum, has come to be called "cooperative adoption."™ In cooperative adoption,™ the child has access to both families, to both sets of parents, and has continuing, progressive participation in the decisions that affect his or her life and relationships. Most open adoptions are not cooperative in the sense of requiring a continuing relationship, but they do encourage some degree of contact over the years so that adoptees can find and know more about their birth parent(s) if and when they want to.

Increasingly, birth mothers who know about private adoption want to choose the adoptive parents and get to know them to some degree. In California and in other states, most public and private agencies and private counselors request or require some level of relationship and contact. If you want to work with these people, you will need to understand why there is such momentum toward opening up the adoption process.

Like most social institutions, adoption is constantly evolving, and recently it has been undergoing something of a revolution. You have to think back to the past to understand the

context in which our present policies and attitudes evolved.
Remember when a pregnancy by an unmarried girl was a
source of such shame and scandal that she had no choice but
to disappear for a while, give up the baby, and then return
pretending nothing had happened? Remember when children
born out of wedlock were illegitimate "bastards," ostracized
if their background became known? Remember when people
whispered that little Fred was adopted behind his back? Remember when infertility was not a household word and couples who adopted felt obligated to keep their child's origin a
secret, at least until the child came of age?

Some of these attitudes still prevail in many parts of the
country, and in most states adoption laws reflect the emphasis
on complete secrecy that has been at the heart of adoption
for over fifty years. Adoption records are sealed, and even
the adopted child cannot get to them without a court order.
Many birth parents and adoptive parents are glad to know
that their privacy is protected. But in urban and suburban
areas nationwide, and particularly in California, the climate
for adoption has changed radically. Many birth mothers now
want to choose the families with whom they place their babies,
and they want to have some future contact with the child, if
only through pictures and letters. Rather than "putting the
child up for adoption," they are "making an adoption plan"
for their child. Adoptive couples are opening up to having a
relationship with the birth parents and extending that relationship to their child or children.

To most people, this "open" approach to adoption seems
crazy and loaded with potential problems. Others feel it is a
change that is long overdue. Like it or not, this is the direction
in which adoption is going—and it is happening rapidly. What
is driving the revolution seems to be a combination of factors
reflecting the experience of various participants in the adoption triangle—birth parents (mostly birth mothers), adoptees,
social workers, and adoptive parents.

The women's movement, having opened up a whole new arena of choices for women, has emboldened both the young women who are now getting pregnant and the older women who gave up their babies for adoption in years past. Women who gave up their babies in the fifties and sixties, often under duress, are lobbying for birth mothers' rights—particularly the right to know where their children are and how they are doing in life. They want the world to know that, contrary to general opinion, they are not uncaring mothers who got rid of their babies and just forgot about them. Rather, they say that they suffer deep and long-lasting feelings of grief and guilt as well as the pain of not knowing what has happened to their children. Birth mothers have formed organizations such as Concerned United Birthparents, with chapters throughout the country, that promote changes in the institution of adoption —particularly giving birth parents more rights and a greater role in the process.

Another source of momentum for open adoption is adoptees who have grown up with their backgrounds hidden from them and who, as adults, are searching out their biological roots. Whether or not they knew they were adopted, and no matter whether their adoptive parents were absolutely ideal, many adoptees want to know about their blood families. Many have gone through grueling, lengthy, and sometimes humiliating searches. They have found the adoption system completely closed to their pleas for help in locating birth parents, and they are outraged that even as adults they do not have access to what they consider to be basic, personal information to which they are entitled. They, too, have formed organizations working for adoption reform and aimed at helping adoptees and birth parents find each other. They believe that reunions with their biological parents are crucial to their psychological well-being, and they want to abolish the system of closed records.

A third force in the growing open adoption movement is

psychologists, counselors, and social workers who work with the participants in the adoption triangle. Many of them recognize the continuing pain of disenfranchised birth parents, and they feel that the closed adoption system has a very negative impact on adoptive children—"the victims of secrecy." According to these professionals, there is a good deal of psychological literature pointing to a disproportionate amount of problems among adoptees, particularly a significantly higher incidence of mental illness and criminal behavior. These problems are attributed to the "object loss" of the natural parents: The adopted child lacks a fundamental aspect of his or her identity. This loss or lack results in continued identity problems and in psychological maladjustment. The cure for these problems is a reunion of the child and the biological family, and the prevention is an adoption process that allows for contact and openness within the adoption triangle.

While concern for the adoptive parents is not the primary focus of the open adoption movement, its advocates claim that this side of the triangle also suffers under the closed system. Adoptive parents may not have all the information they would like or might need in the future about their child. Those who have not worked through their infertility may feel they are not really entitled to have a child, and their behavior as parents may suffer. According to Dr. Arthur Sorosky, Annette Baran, and Reuben Pannor, the authors of *The Adoption Triangle*, a landmark book in promoting open adoption, adoptive parents as a rule have real problems in parenting. While they are not likely to take their children for granted, says the book, "as a group, adoptive parents are insecure in their role as parents and tend to be overprotective of their children. They are often overindulgent, overpermissive, and disinclined to exert effective discipline. These behaviors are an overcompensation to prove they are good parents." They also have "perfectionistic expectations of their children" and, if the child does not live up to them, they attribute behavioral difficulties to heredity, that is, the child's "bad blood." A more open adoption process, say the advocates, allows adoptive parents to understand and deal more effectively with their children and recognize the special needs of the adoptive family. It frees them to be honest and forthright with their children and to give them the fullest possible experience of their identity and origins. Open adoption, its advocates claim, is a process in which no one loses and everyone wins.

When I first began to read and talk with adoption counselors about the pressures building toward open adoption, I was frankly astonished at the picture painted of the closed adoption process. It all sounded like the makings of a first-rate soap opera: the adoptive family considered a hotbed of potential maladjustment; aggrieved birth mothers fighting for their rights; adoptees who believe they can never feel whole until they meet or know about their biological parents; and social workers and counselors dedicated to changing the system, becoming advocates for birth parents or even supporting them in keeping their babies rather than giving them up for adoption.

All of this seems to add up to a real nightmare for people who want to adopt. They have visions, as Bill and I did, of having to adopt a teenage mother as well as her child. They see social workers who are at best suspicious of them and at worst hostile to their interests. They see birth mothers wanting to reclaim babies after a few months or never really giving them up—wanting to babysit every weekend, buy them clothes, or spend Christmas and Mothers Day with them. They see children confused and conflicted about which mommy is which and why they have two. They see themselves, desperate survivors of their war with infertility, entering another war of fighting to be seen as the "real" parents of their child. And because they are so desperate, they see themselves forced to tolerate situations they would not choose and do not want.

Fortunately, according to the participants, the reality of open adoption does not seem to bear out all of these fears. Seeking some answers about the issues involved in open adoption, I talked with a number of adoptive couples and with adoption lawyers, counselors, and social workers representing the spectrum of opinion and practice.

Philip Adams,* the California lawyer who handled our adoption of Alexander, has been the attorney for thousands of adoptions over the past forty years. He began arranging for clients to meet each other as early as 1950, having noticed that many privately arranged "hand to hand" adoptions in which people knew each other seemed to go quite well. Over the years, he has encouraged people to get to know each other before the birth, and he has seen an increasing trend for that relationship to continue after the adoption. He feels the deep dark secrecy of adoption is an anachronism, and although he doesn't require open adoptions, he has found that adoptive couples end up enthusiastic about it, "almost in inverse proportion to the degree of their resistance to it beforehand."

Bruce Rappaport is director of the Independent Adoption Center, a nonprofit organization that has handled over 300 private adoptions here in the San Franscisco Bay Area between 1982 and 1988. Bruce prefers to call open adoption "normalized adoption," partly because the other term sounds too much like "open marriage" (and carries its unorthodox connotations), and partly because "normalized" is really a more accurate term. It is *normal* for people who are engaged in such an important personal process to know each other's names, meet each other, and have normal, human contact. The Independent Adoption Center helps birth parents and adoptive parents find each other and meet each other. It counsels both parties about adoption and serves as a mediator if there are any conflicts or problems. The key to a successful open

---

*I have used the real names of adoption professionals in this chapter.

adoption, says Rappaport, is a good match of adoptive couple and birth parent(s) and the agreement of both parties as to the type and degree of relationship they want. Problems arise when any party is not honest or open about what he or she wants and tries to change the arrangement after the fact.

Bruce Rappaport is anything but dogmatic about the adoption process, and his organization will handle any type of adoption. But he finds that when people resist openness, it is usually out of fear and misinformation. He says that a birth mother who does not want to know about the adoptive parents is usually ashamed about giving up her baby and feels she is doing something wrong. When she receives counseling and starts to believe she is doing something good and honorable, she usually wants to meet the couple. An adoptive couple resisting openness usually comes to recognize that they want a birth mother who cares about her baby, and generally they agree that that kind of mother would want to have a say in her baby's future. Bruce poses the question to them: If you were 18 and pregnant and knew you had a choice, would you want to choose your baby's future family? Most couples honestly have to answer yes. Bruce's experience is that most couples who adopt this way end up appreciating and even treasuring their relationship with the birth parent(s). Rather than hearing complaints from parents about too much birth mother contact, he hears the opposite—"We don't hear from Karen often enough. Do you have an address for us?" (The Independent Adoption Center does request that its birth mothers keep them informed of their whereabouts, but not all do.)

Other open adoption advocates are far more adamant about the need for contact and relationship. Ellen Curtis is a lay adoption counselor who lives in Marin County, California, but has clients throughout the country. She is the mother of three daughters, two adopted and one biological, all born within a year. She herself was adopted by a stepparent, and her husband, a physician, has a birth son now in his twenties. In this living adoption laboratory, Ellen has evolved into a strong proponent of cooperative adoption—maintaining a lifelong relationship between biological and adoptive families. Both her adoptions were initially closed, but one of her daughters exhibited emotional problems at age 4 that Ellen began to recognize as adoption-related. After working with others in the adoption field and solving problems with both adoptees and their parents, Ellen decided to locate both her daughters' birth parents and establish relationships with them.

It took Ellen three or four years of careful courting to get the two sets of birth mothers and their families interested in connecting with her and their birth children. Their reluctance, Ellen feels, stemmed from their own grief and denial—a situation that needed to be healed. Ellen's overtures finally paid off, and one extraordinary Christmas a few years ago, the Curtis family heard from both sets of birth parents and also from the grown birth son. They are all now a part of the extended Curtis family, considered as close relatives with mutual visits occurring several times a year. One Curtis daughter was the flower girl in her birth mother's wedding.

Ellen Curtis's Cooperative Adoption Service is aimed at preparing parents for what she says are those 50 percent of adoptions in which the child is at high risk of emotional problems. While many adoptive children suffer no psychological problems and have little concern about their biological roots, just as many have feelings of rejection and abandonment that simply cannot be loved away. These are the children who end up, in disproportionate numbers, in the juvenile and psychiatric systems. Cooperative adoption is aimed at preventing or alleviating such problems. Ellen reports that her problem daughter is now "a fuller, more rounded person" and far happier now that she knows her birth mother. Her adoption clients, whom she asks for continuing information about their experience, report that their relationships are valuable and rewarding. Again, the adoptive parents complain of too little rather than too much contact with the birth parents.

Of course, the practice of having a familial relationship with birth parents is not new. Throughout history, children have been adopted by aunts and uncles, sisters and brothers, grandparents, and even close family friends. But cooperative adoption among people who are not friends or family is too new for there to be scientific data on its effects—whether it does indeed solve problems or, as critics charge, creates them. Some adoption professionals and many adoptive couples worry about the long-term effect on the children and about people feeling pressured to be involved in relationships they don't want to have. The Independent Adoption Center, for example, has not moved toward the cooperative adoption end of the spectrum. Although it works well for some people, Bruce Rappaport feels it often makes the birth mother feel guilty for not wanting to maintain a lifelong relationship with her child.

While open and cooperative adoption thrives in California's more freewheeling social climate, it has not yet found fertile ground elsewhere. In Oklahoma, for example, our beloved Scott Roberts still finds birth mothers who prefer not to know the people who adopt their offspring and who say they do not want contact with them after their babies are born. Scott has handled more than one hundred and fifty adoptions over the past thirty years and disagrees with just about everything the open adoption advocates are pushing. His perspective, shared by most of the couples in his California network, provides another side of the open adoption question. He feels open adoption and open adoption records encourage problems by invading people's privacy and pressuring people into relationships they do not want. He feels children need only one set of parents and do not need the confusion of trying to distinguish and relate to more than one mom or dad. He does not see any evidence of an abnormal amount of maladjustment among the children he has placed.

Scott does not corroborate the reports of continuing angst and grief among birth mothers. He says the young women whose babies he has placed do not come back to him asking questions or wanting contact. When he sees them years later, they do not inquire about their children. They are happy to have that part of their lives behind them and to get on with living, usually marrying and having other children. Most have specifically asked to have the baby go out of state so they know they won't run into him or her on the street some day. They would not take kindly, he says, to a birth child's showing up on their doorstep, possibly embarrassing them or causing problems for their families. He feels it is best for everyone that Oklahoma's birth records are sealed and that it would take a court order for anyone to find out the birth parents' names. Open adoption, he believes, not only makes for uncomfortable and unnecessary intrusions into people's family lives, it also encourages the birth mother not to completely let go of the child.

Scott Roberts is particularly exasperated by social workers, "meddling do-gooders" who he feels sow the seeds of doubt in birth mothers' minds about giving up the baby. "If you ask someone again and again if they are sure they are doing the right thing," he says, "they are bound to start questioning themselves." In his thirty-year career, only four birth mothers have changed their minds at the last minute, but none have taken back babies they already relinquished. In the latest case, the mother was quite clear about her decision (she was on welfare and already had one child with severe medical problems) until a social worker at the hospital insisted she keep her newborn baby with her overnight. The next morning she was hysterical, screaming that she could not give up her child. Scott feels all parties—the mother, the disappointed couple, and the baby—suffer from such insensitive intervention. With his California clients, Scott carefully fends off social workers trying to contact birth parents about adoptions that are already final in Oklahoma. "If they had their way," he says, "they'd try to talk them into taking back the babies."

Fear of a baby's being reclaimed is at the heart of most people's concerns about open adoption. Most of us assume that once the birth mother sees and spends any time with her baby, she will want to keep him or her. Although a change of heart and mind is rare, Philip Adams recognizes that possibility and advises his clients to put off a visit by the birth mother until after the consent to adoption papers have been signed. Other adoption professionals say that open adoption decreases the chances for a failed adoption, that when a birth mother has a personal relationship with the adoptive couple, she is less likely to change her mind. Bruce Rappaport of the Independent Adoption Center says only 1 to 2 percent of his adoptions have ended this way, and usually only because adoptive parents reneged on the agreements they made with the birth mother for contact after the baby was born.

Bruce Rappaport, Ellen Curtis, and other professionals see a very important result of open adoption that most of us might not recognize. They think that it will increase the number of babies available for adoption. Many birth mothers choose to have an abortion or to keep a child rather than turn it over to an agency and never know what becomes of it. Once they know they can create an adoption plan for their child and maintain some level of contact, they feel more comfortable about choosing that option. Part of the work of the Independent Adoption Center is an outreach program to inform pregnant young women about the choices they have. Surprisingly, the IAC has met with resistance from some women's organizations who categorize them as "pro-lifers" trying to prevent abortions. They find that family planning counselors are often afraid of or resistant to giving out adoption information. Bruce Rappaport hopes that women's organizations and pro-choice advocates will come to recognize that promoting adoption is not antifeminist. It is not a threat to a woman's choice, but rather an expansion of that choice, as well as a potential blessing for the millions of couples who seek to adopt a child.

The picture the professionals paint of open adoption is a fairly rosy one, and for the most part it is borne out by adoptive couples. Most of the couples I talked to were initially resistant and afraid, but as they got to know their birth mother as a person, their fears dissipated and they were grateful for the experience. Doug and Carolyn found out about a birth mother in West Virginia through adoption counselors Bonnie and Marc Gradstein, lawyers who run a private adoption service in Northern California. Bobbie, the birth mother, was anxious to get away from a bad home situation, and Doug and Carolyn agreed to pay her way to California to meet them. She would then go on to live with her father in Southern California during her pregnancy.

Doug and Carolyn were very nervous about meeting Bobbie, but they got along well with her. They were also happy when she reassured them several times that she would not change her mind and keep the baby. In the months that followed, they visited her once at her father's home, and they were present at the hospital for the birth. Ecstatic that baby Elizabeth was now theirs, they felt great love and gratitude toward Bobbie but hoped she would keep her distance a bit during their early weeks of being a family. In fact, Bobbie did not visit them or see her daughter again, though Carolyn sent her pictures every few months. In return, she received a couple of very lovely letters from Bobbie expressing her happiness that Elizabeth was with such a good family and her sadness that she was not able to keep her. The communication by letters continues, and Carolyn keeps them so that in the future Elizabeth can know a little about her birth mother should she choose to.

Several other couples I talked with had similar experiences with their birth mothers (no one had birth fathers involved), and some had more extensive contact. Eve and George invited their birth mother to live with them for several months prior to birth and then served as her labor coaches. Once the girl moved away, they kept in contact by phone, but they find the number of times they talk is diminishing.

There are those couples who wish for less contact with the birth mother, however. Ever since their child was born, Fred and Sarah have been visited by their birth mother, Lydia, about once a week. Lately, she has asked them if she can take the baby to visit her family, a large Latino clan. Sarah and George are nervous and unhappy but haven't found the courage to tell her no. They feel so grateful for the gift she gave them that they find it difficult to draw the line. Kelley and Ben's birth mother, Teresa, lived with them for two months before the birth and has returned to visit two or three times since. This past Christmas, when Teresa stayed with them for almost two weeks, they were extremely uncomfortable. It seems their 1-year-old daughter Kim grew very attached to her birth mother, wanting to spend all her time with Teresa and rejecting Kelley, who was heartbroken. Both of these situations point up the need not only for all parties to be clear in advance what kind of relationship they want, but also to be able to express themselves openly and honestly as the relationship progresses.

Most birth mothers in open adoptions do not want the kind of contact that Lydia and Teresa want. Many feel it is wrong—confusing to the child and possibly undermining the adoptive parents—and many just want to focus on their own lives. They appreciate, however, that they know who their child is with, that they were able to choose his or her family, that they can communicate with the child if necessary and at the least see pictures over time. The few birth mothers I talked to were grateful that their adoptions did not occur in a shroud of secrecy but were not anxious to be a part of their children's lives.

Carrie, now 22, placed her daughter with a family in another state specifically so she could maintain her distance. She loved knowing her daughter was all right and seeing pictures of her as she grew up, but she felt it would be bad to confuse her with "two mothers." She wrote a long letter to her daughter explaining why she had had to give her up and asked that the mother read it to her when she was ready.

While the results of open adoptions may be beneficial, the process is not always easy. It is certainly more demanding emotionally than just receiving a baby with no real live person involved and no strings attached. In an open adoption, the relationship between adoptive parents and birth mother can be a very intense one, and the transfer of the baby into its new family is not always completely smooth. Our friends Martin and Sylvia spent two very emotional days with their birth mother, a 16-year-old named Karen, immediately after Jason was born. At first giddy and excited after a very easy birth, within hours Karen grew extremely sad and depressed about letting go of her child and about the fact that her own mother had refused to come be with her at the birth. Martin and Sylvia, fearful about the outcome of the adoption, were equally upset. They spent many anxious hours at the hospital talking to Karen, listening to her concerns and fears, and trying to give her emotional support. It was two days and two sleepless nights before she re-resolved to go through with the adoption and they were able to take their baby home with them. But despite the excruciating fear and sadness of those forty-eight hours, Martin and Sylvia are grateful to have known Karen and to have been able to be there for her. "She endured a lot to give us our son," they said. "We were glad to be able to give something back." They also felt that if they had not known Karen and could not have given her the support she needed, she very possibly would have changed her mind and kept the baby.

In comparison to our friends' experience, our closed adoption was easy and delightful. After the birth, we had only baby Alexander to worry about and did not really know what Eileen might be experiencing. Still, after talking with adoptive parents, birth mothers, and adoption counselors, I found myself much more favorable toward open adoption, particularly toward people meeting each other. While I don't know what the long-term impact of cooperative adoption will be, it is apparent that some people find it highly appropriate and rewarding. When the fears and shame and self-protection are swept aside, it does make sense for the participants in such an awesome process to at least know and like each other and to have the opportunity to stay in communication. I continue to think of Eileen frequently and wonder if we will ever communicate, if we will ever seek each other out, or if some day Alexander will want us to open up our adoption.

Clearly, adoption is evolving in the direction of openness, but it is important to recognize that it is a highly personal experience and that we still need a range of options tailored not to an ideology, but to the people involved. What is truly unfortunate is that birth mothers or adoptive parents may feel they have no choice in the matter—that they may be pressured by their own fears or by other people to do something that doesn't feel right to them.

One of the major objections to private adoption is that very often couples have to deal with this issue and others without benefit of counseling. Adoption agencies, both public and private, feel adoptive couples as well as birth parents should engage in counseling before and during the adoption process. Counselors Bruce Rappaport and Ellen Curtis believe it is important to make sure that couples are aware of and prepared for issues or problems that may arise in the process. On the other hand, attorneys Philip Adams and Scott Roberts scoff at the idea that adoption participants have to be counseled any more than natural parents do. It may be appropriate or even necessary for some people, especially if problems arise, but plenty of successful adoptions take place without it.

Even though the vast majority of adoptions work out wonderfully for everyone involved, adoption is still a difficult and risky process. Waiting for a baby to adopt can be as stressful and scary as waiting to conceive. And, as with bearing a child, there are no guarantees. A rejection by a birth mother may feel like yet another failure and proof of your inadequacy. A lost lead to a baby may feel like a miscarriage. A child reclaimed can be as devastating as a death. If everything works out, as it usually does, the end reward is, of course, immeasurably wonderful. But the adoption process itself can yield its own rewards. Seeking a child through private adoption or going through an agency home study can be beneficial to your emotional state and to your marriage. After years of feeling completely helpless about trying to get pregnant, here at last is a situation you can do something about. You know that your time and energy can pay off, and you begin to regain a sense of control over your life. While the burden of infertility treatment most often falls on the woman, adoption is something you and your spouse can pursue together. It enables you to work toward a common goal, to feel a sense of purpose, and to again take charge of planning your family's future.

Whatever obstacles you encounter in adopting—a difficult social worker, an unstable birth mother, miscommunication, or a long wait for the right situation—it is important that you keep a positive attitude and try not to get desperate. Desperation breeds bad judgment and bad decisions. Yes, babies are scarce, but not that scarce. If the first adoption situation does not suit you, wait for one that does. If you find a birth mother who wants to babysit every weekend and that's something you won't feel comfortable with, find another one whose contact preferences are closer to yours. Try to keep in mind that you deserve the child and the situation you want. You are not a beggar, but a chooser. There is a child is out there for you—maybe two or three of them. If you are willing to work for it, you *will* have your family!

Part Three

Chapter Nine

❦

Still Trying

*T*here is an old saying, "God makes first babies so good so that you'll have a second one." To us, our son was beyond good, he was Alexander the Great! He increased his adorable quotient even as he became more active and exploratory. All boy, he was fascinated by tools and anything with wheels on it (trucks are his life). He has that genetic trait possessed only by males of the species that enables them to make motor "vrooming" sounds even before they can say their first words. During Alexander's first year, Bill and I lived in a state of "overwhelmment" (I began this book, his construction business was booming), which culminated in our moving out of our house for six months so we could remodel and build an addition for much needed space.

Obviously, we didn't give much thought to having a second child. Both of us felt we wanted another (a little girl, please), but we simply assumed that if we didn't get pregnant we would adopt again through Scott Roberts. Although we continued to make love without birth control, we were actually relieved that we didn't suddenly become fertile, as everyone had assured us we would. But as our house began to take shape, and as Alexander grew into toddlerhood and I grew deeper into my forties, I began to think a lot about baby number two. It would be best, I felt, if she came along about the time Alexander was 3. But I would be 45 then, and as young as I looked and felt, I could not escape visions of someone asking my daughter, "Is that your grandmother?"

Given our wonderful experience with Alexander, I felt positive about adopting again, but I found it hard to imagine that we could be as lucky the second time as we were the first. Our boy had turned out to be so beautiful, happy, and healthy—did we dare hope for a child such as he again? Bill was also happy about the prospect of adopting another child and continued to talk about trying a foreign adoption. I started to get interested in that idea as well. Since I didn't feel the same pressure now, maybe it would be easier to deal with the wait and the hassles.

I can't say that I gave up on the biological route, however. When I met a woman chiropractor whom I liked a lot and who claimed to have had several patients who got pregnant after lower back treatment, I decided to be treated myself. Her manipulations helped my back, for which I was grateful, but that was all. I also bought one of those ovulation predictor kits and played junior chemist, mixing vials of whatever it was and watching pieces of white paper turn blue. Invariably, I'd forget about the correct timing of each sequence, so I was never quite sure about the results. Even when I did it right, it still didn't work. Slowly, I began to accept that I might never bear a child in this lifetime. The thought saddened me, but I was so happy with Alexander and my life was so full of activity and love that I didn't dwell on it.

Meanwhile, I was steeped in the process of writing this

book, and a friend told me about a fertility specialist he knew
in Phoenix who was having phenomenal results with his patients. I called Dr. Jay Nemiro* of the Arizona Center for Fertility Studies and in a brief conversation got very interested
in exploring his approach and results for this book. Fortunately, I was able to meet him in San Francisco for an interview
a few weeks later.

Dark, handsome, and intensely energetic, Dr. Nemiro
talked for a couple of hours about his work with the excitement of a man with a mission. In fact, he does have a commitment "to end infertility by the year 2000." Here and now,
that commitment translates into a very aggressive treatment
strategy—doing something that works, quickly and efficiently.
For starters, he tells his patients to throw their thermometers
against the wall ("No one ever got pregnant taking their temperature") and move on to something that can result in pregnancy, even if it may be inconvenient and more expensive. For
the most part, "what works" for Jay Nemiro is his version of
GIFT, called Low Tubal Transfer, or LTT. Conceptually, the
procedure is the same as GIFT, but because of differences in
his technique, he prefers his own terminology.

LTT was developed in 1984 by Dr. Nemiro and his partner, Dr. Robert McGaughey, a scientist and professor who
specializes in reproductive biology. Frustrated with the poor
results and high cost of in vitro fertilization, they sat one morning at "The Good Egg" restaurant in Phoenix and worked out
a protocol for their first low tubal transfers. Like GIFT, LTT
involves using fertility drugs to stimulate the production of
many eggs, retrieving the eggs through a laparoscopy, and then
mixing the eggs with prepared sperm and injecting the mixture
directly into the fallopian tube, where fertilization naturally
takes place. A woman must have at least one open tube, but
eggs are not required—Dr. Nemiro will use donor eggs if nec-

---

*His real name.

essary. Over the past four years the Nemiro-McGaughey team has refined the LTT technique to the point that 52 percent of their patients get pregnant, resulting in a 38 percent live birth rate (the 24 percent miscarriage rate is fairly normal). Given that most GIFT programs claim only a 15 to 30 percent live birth rate, these guys seem to be doing something right. Also, their charge for the operation in 1988 was $2800 to $3000— less than half the cost of IVF and substantially less than most GIFT programs.

It was not just his success rate that impressed me about Dr. Nemiro, however; it was his intense "go for it" attitude and his personal commitment "to leave no stone unturned to get you pregnant—and fast." Some couples, particularly in the early stages of treatment, are put off by such aggressiveness, but many veterans of the infertility war are thrilled to find a doctor who is as militant as they are. In our case, for example, Dr. Nemiro said he would not have waited for six unsuccessful intrauterine inseminations before doing a laparoscopy but would have suggested it early on. And rather than doing just an exploratory laparoscopy, he routinely prepares the patient for the LTT procedure at the same time. If he finds the tubes are damaged, he will do the necessary surgery, but if he finds at least one is intact, he can then proceed with the LTT. "If you're going to pay for an operation," he said, "why not do something that can result in pregnancy?"

I could appreciate the doctor's direct approach and his success, but it seemed a little too good to be true. I asked questions to try to find some holes in his story. What about the high incidence of multiple births? Because he routinely uses five or more eggs in the procedure, many of his patients end up with two or more babies. Most GIFT and IVF programs report a 20 percent chance of multiple births, but the LTT seems to have spawned more than its share of twins, triplets, and even quadruplets—about 32 percent of births have been multiple (90 percent twins, but also triplets and quadruplets).

Nemiro, father of four children, was nonchalant about the multiple births. He tells his patients, "All of you are taking the chances for each other," and, he said, they are willing to do it. Who are his patients? They are mostly couples in their early thirties with unexplained infertility. Does he exclude women over 40? He said that he has had a number of patients in their forties and that he would work with women over 45 if other factors were in place. (Recently a 47-year-old patient became pregnant with triplets as a result of using donor eggs.) Dr. Nemiro said his results are about the same with older patients as with younger ones. What about miscarriage? Over the past year, he began prescribing daily shots of progesterone for two weeks following the LTT and found it reduces the miscarriage rate from 30 percent to 24 percent—below the norm for GIFT and IVF programs. To what does he attribute his success? He said that since he and his partner are constantly refining the variables of LTT they will continue to improve their success rate. He did not believe there was some magic number above which the rate could not rise.

I left my interview with Dr. Nemiro impressed and somewhat agitated. I hadn't intended to think about any more fertility treatment, but I found myself considering the operation and almost a 40 percent chance to produce a baby. Maybe it would be less because of my age, but the chances were still good. When I told Bill about my interview and Dr. Nemiro's success with the LTT, he was less than enthusiastic. He was still concerned about what pregnancy would do to me and felt it would be easier and more cost effective to pursue another adoption. I wasn't ready myself to take on yet another project, so I dropped the matter for a while.

A few weeks later, we had adoption on our minds again as the biannual visit of Scott and Margaret Roberts from Oklahoma brought together the entire California network of adoptive families. We began what would turn into a week's worth of festivities with the annual picnic at Marie and Carl's house, a wild event made wilder this year by trying to get a photo portrait of Scott and Margaret and all their "godchildren." Cameras clicked and whirred as babies screamed, toddlers squirmed, and 6-year-olds punched each other. Just as we finally wriggled Alexander into the picture, little Lacey would run out. Kids kept replacing each other as fast as we could gather them, so the ordeal continued for at least half an hour.

There was also time for getting to know the other couples, admiring their kids—"Looks just like you!"—and swapping stories. The most heartbreaking was of one couple who had pursued an adoption of a second child on their own here in California. They met the birth mother, had lunch with her, and felt wonderful about the situation. But just before the baby was to be born, the young woman called and said she had changed her mind because they had had a glass of wine with lunch. She had decided they would not be proper parents for her child. The couple was stunned. There were much happier stories: One of the adoptive mothers had just had a "miracle baby" (doctors said she had one chance in a million to get pregnant) and another had also just given birth. Biological babies had come to a few other adoptive moms over the years, but generally the group did not provide evidence for the "Adopt and then you'll get pregant" doctrine. A few couples had adopted two children through Scott, and, it became apparent, a lot more were planning on it. Talking to all the other mothers who were considering number two, I felt sort of panicky. Would Scott find enough babies to go around? I figured I'd better let him know right away we were interested.

We spent a couple of evenings with the Robertses over the next week, listening to all of Scott's adoption stories, some funny, some hair-raising—for instance, the girl who came in to the hospital to have her baby in the morning and by afternoon had contacted him, signed the papers, and relinquished the child because she had to be home by 5 P.M. or her parents would punish her. Evidently, they had had no idea she was pregnant. Then there was the fundamentalist group who came around to the hospital to try to talk a teenage girl into keeping her baby. Scott said it was a great idea; would they be willing to sign papers stating that they would all help support her and the baby financially? The group made a hasty exit.

The adoptive couples all had their stories, too; it seems the trip to Tulsa was as mind-blowing for other couples as it had been for us. Tornadoes prevented Beverly and David's plane from taking off. Joe and Elaine got treated to a luncheon with the judge and the chief of police that featured a lingerie show. Several couples had unforgettable tours of the Cowboy Museum, and many were outfitted with cowboy hats at Scott's favorite haberdashery. Everyone raved about how wonderfully they'd been taken care of by the Robertses. This week in California was our opportunity to return the hospitality, and the Robertses were booked for breakfast, lunch, and dinner all over the Bay Area.

At a banquet (without kids) the final night of their stay, toasts flowed and there was not a dry eye in the room. Since the couples present did not know their birth mothers, we had only Scott Roberts to thank for the most precious gift ever to come into our lives. We let our gratitude pour out in a sort of "love feast" honoring Scott, Margaret, and Philip Adams, our California attorney. I wished that night that all the young women who had given of their flesh and blood could have known and felt what a difference they had made in our lives. I hoped the energy of our love and gratitude would somehow touch their hearts and heal any sadness or regret. I thought of Eileen and how proud she would be of having had such a sweet, handsome boy.

I had come to feel much more positive toward open adoption—at least toward having some contact with the birth mother—and was somewhat sad that Scott Roberts was against it. That didn't stop me, however, from letting Scott know that Bill and I were interested in adopting another baby

through him soon. He said he'd be happy to oblige us but let
us know that we were about eighth on his list—behind some
new referrals and other couples who wanted second children.
We were shocked and disappointed to realize our "sure thing"
could take a couple of years—perhaps shorter but maybe
longer. I began to think about other adoption alternatives, but
the prospect of a massive letter-writing campaign left me cold.
I could not imagine taking on such a project while trying to
finish the book and our house.

Meanwhile, my mind would not let go of the thought of
making one last effort to bear a child. I called Dr. Nemiro for
more information about LTT. He was encouraging and recommended that, given my age, I should do it as soon as
possible. I also talked to our specialist, Dr. B, who was reassuring about the multiple birth problem. If there were more
than two embryos, I could have what is euphemistically called
a "reduction." If we were prepared to do what is essentially
a very early abortion, we would not have to have more than
two babies. With this reassurance, I was ready to talk again
to Bill.

He hadn't wanted to think about it, he said, hoping the
issue would go away for a while. He hoped that we could wait
a couple of years and then get a girl through adoption. But
wouldn't he like to have a little MaryBill? He said he would
like to have a biological child but was afraid to consider more
fertility treatment and the prospect of getting back into the
hope/disappointment syndrome. He also wondered if he
would feel any differently toward a biological child than he
did toward Alexander. Could it be a problem to have one
adopted and one biological child? He again raised his fears
about what pregnancy would do to me physically, about
Down's syndrome, and about multiple births, but it seemed
that something had changed. If having our baby was that important to me, he would go along with one last try. He promised support but not enthusiasm, and I promised him that we

would only do the operation once. The next day, I called Dr. Nemiro about coming to Phoenix in August for the LTT procedure.

As the operation date grew closer, my feet got colder. Having just attended my twenty-fifth high school reunion in North Carolina, I was acutely aware of my age, but I just didn't feel ready yet. The house and the book were pressing on me, and I decided to put off the operation until September, and then October. But in October we were homeless nomads; our rental house lease was up and our renovated house wouldn't be ready for another month. We were staying in friends' houses amidst much chaos—wait until November. In November we moved into a construction zone. More chaos and stress—wait until December. I knew if I didn't decide to take the plunge this year, I would probably not make it. In March I would turn 44, just too close to 45 for comfort. In my mind, age 45 was a sort of a cutoff point, the moment the biological clock would strike midnight and Cinderella would have to leave the ball.

Feeling the pressure to decide, I began to question whether I really wanted another child. Alexander was so real and present, so completely demanding and enthralling. Number two was an abstraction, something I wanted "out there," not something I really craved right now as I had craved number one. And didn't everyone tell me that one and one don't add up to two, that there is something exponential at work in having another child—all systems multiplied by at least two squared? And what if I had twins? My mind boggled at the calculations. Still, our happy family of three didn't feel complete. Both Bill and I had siblings and knew their joys and horrors. We still felt our boy should have a little brother or sister to love and hate.

In late November, I began making the preparations for the operation, meeting with Dr. B here to get the Pergonal and Clomid, trying to make reservations to Phoenix based on the schedule of my cycle—"Yes, I'd like the morning flight on day nine, please." In fact, I did have to be there on day 9 for an ultrasound to see how the eggs were developing, and then Bill would fly in the day before the operation (probably day 13 or 14) to do his part. As the time approached, I found myself feeling not excitement, but fear, anxiety, and sadness. Just walking back into Dr. B's office after almost two years brought up the familiar feel of the fertility roller-coaster ride. Why was I putting myself through this again?

One night, my anxiety came to a head during a conversation with Bill about how hard he was working and how much pressure he felt in our lives. Somehow I ended up yelling and hitting him, screaming about the pressure I was under and how alone I felt in pursuing the operation. I hadn't realized until I became half-hysterical what a burden it was to feel that Bill wasn't really behind this attempt at having a biological baby. "Why don't you just tell me no, you won't do it! Are you going to wait until we have twins and then just leave me?" As I sobbed into the pillows of our bed, Bill held me and stroked me. He told me how sorry he was and that he hadn't realized how alone I felt. Yes, despite all his doubts and fears, he did want me to get pregnant and he would support me completely throughout the process. I would not have to go through this alone. All the pent-up tension of the past months seemed to let go. I knew he was telling the truth, that he would be there for me, and at that moment I felt I loved him more than was humanly possible.

Feeling I had a partner again made me feel much better about undergoing daily shots of Pergonal, that very expensive fertility drug that Dr. B told us "comes from the urine of post-menopausal Italian nuns." We thought he was joking, but it turns out that the hormone is distilled from human female urine and that Serono Laboratories in Italy has the exclusive patent on it. Bill joked that he hoped I wouldn't start saying "Hail Marys." Bill would be administering the daily shots, and since we were both nervous the first time, we had a friend who was a nurse help us out. The glass vials and needles were intimidating, but actually the process was fairly simple. In a few days, Bill felt like a pro. I felt no side effects from the Pergonal, nor were the shots painful. Still, getting a shot in the butt is not the greatest way to wake up in the morning. Now, the issue was how I would respond. How many of my eggs would come out for this occasion? I looked forward to a whole Easter basketfull.

On Day 7, I had my first ultrasound, now done intra-vaginally—an improvement over the water torture method. There were only four eggs present, two on each side, and only one was "good-sized." At first I thought this was fine, that four was plenty, but when I spoke with Dr. Nemiro on the phone a few minutes later, he said he had hoped for a better response—at least four or five good ones to transfer into the tubes. If all four of these eggs grew appreciably, we might be able to go ahead, but we might have to wait and try again with a different drug protocol next month. He didn't want to decide now but would await the results of another ultrasound, preferably on Saturday. My heart tumbled to the floor of the radiologist's office. The thought of aborting this mission stunned me.

Driving back across the Golden Gate Bridge in the bright winter sun, the situation began to sink in and I felt old and inadequate. I had not even considered that I would not respond to the Pergonal. Maybe Dr. A, my gynecologist, was right: My little egg nests, which had been producing monthly since age 11, just might be nearing the end of their supply. I was becoming barren. At home I moped around, unable to work. When I looked in the mirror, all I could see was the silver overtaking the blonde in my hair and lines tracing my features even when I wasn't smiling.

Radiologists don't work on ovulation time, meaning I couldn't find anyone to do the ultrasound on Saturday and had to go in Friday afternoon. Only three of the eggs had grown, and only one of those was large enough to qualify as "good-sized." Dr. Nemiro's nurse advised me on the phone that we would not be going ahead with the operation. Dr. Nemiro was out of town but would talk to me next week about trying again next month. The familiarity of the disappointment did not make it any easier. I fought back tears as I called Dr. B's office. I realized I could at least have another intrauterine insemination, which I scheduled with him for Monday morning. That night I drank a few glasses of wine, cried on Bill's shoulder, and called my friends to tell them I wouldn't be going to Phoenix. Telling people "I didn't make enough eggs" made me feel like a worn-out old hen.

Over the weekend, I felt subdued and somewhat sad, but it was hard to stay depressed around irrepressible Alexander. That boy could charm the blues out of the sky. By Monday, I was even feeling a little hopeful about the IUI (lucky number seven?), but after the procedure, I felt the familiar fear of hoping once again. I did not hope for long. When my period arrived several days early and lasted only three days, I began to wonder if I was entering the early stages of menopause. Despite my discouragement, Dr. Nemiro was still encouraging, letting me know that we could try again right away with a new fertility drug, Lupron, which is sometimes successful in women who don't respond to Pergonal alone. Sometimes, he told me, a woman's own body signals interfere with the effects of the Pergonal, and Lupron, a hormone administered in the two weeks before the Pergonal cycle, shuts down those signals, essentially creating a "false menopause." With no stimulation to interfere, the Pergonal cycle can then be completely controlled. The next step for me would be to try this drug protocol or to go with the option he felt held the most promise—donor eggs.

The idea of getting pregnant with another woman's eggs did not immediately appeal to me, but I listened as he explained the process. Probably the main factor in my infertility was the age of my eggs, and he had found that using the eggs of a younger woman (preferably in her twenties) greatly increased the chances of the LTT's success. We could ask someone we knew to donate her eggs, or we could use the extra eggs produced by one of his other LTT patients. Some women respond to Pergonal by producing as many as ten or fifteen eggs and have a few good ones to spare. If we did choose to go with one of his patients, we would not be able to specify any physical characteristics of the donor—the choice would be his based on the timing of his procedures. He would pick a month when there were many operations scheduled, and we would come to Phoenix to await "appropriate eggs." If we found our own egg donor, the logistics would also be complex. She would need to undergo the Pergonal regimen at the same time that I was treated with Lupron to prepare me for the LTT.

The donor egg scenario sounded a bit bizarre to me, but I discussed it with Bill. We started fantasizing about who we might enroll as an egg donor. Most of our friends were too old, but perhaps one of my nieces.... They were both young, gorgeous, intelligent, and talented. But they were both in college and unlikely to have much time for shots and tests and trips to Phoenix. And how would they feel about being both cousin and mom?

Before we continued with that line of investigation, we felt we should look further into the chances of my making my own eggs. But with the past month's disappointment still weighing on me and the Christmas holidays approaching, I was not in much of a frame of mind for decision making. The issue was tabled until after New Year's.

My number-one resolution for the new year was to have baby number two—one way or the other. I knew what my options were: to try Pergonal and Lupron in hopes of making my own eggs for the LTT; to go ahead with the LTT with donor eggs, either from friend, relative, or stranger; or to pursue finding a baby through adoption. It seemed highly unlikely that we would get a baby through Scott Roberts any time in the next year. We were still eighth on the list and Scott was having a drought of sorts. Unless something remarkable happened, we could not expect another baby from Oklahoma in the next twelve months. But if the options before me were clear, what I wanted was not. I knew the decision was mine and that Bill would support me whatever my choice, but I felt entirely confused.

How much did I really want to bear our own (or at least Bill's) child? What was I willing to go through to do it? I knew I could handle the disappointment if further fertility treatment didn't work—that I was used to. But what if treatment did work? What would it be like to be pregnant and have a 2-year-old at age 44 or 45? What if I ended up with twins or triplets? What if I went through all the trouble and expense and had a miscarriage? How would I cope with the pain? How attached was I to the experience of pregnancy and giving birth? Most women I knew did not rave about the joys of being pregnant, and few would choose childbirth—aside from its outcome—as an experience they would repeat. Did these concerns make sense, or was I just afraid? I remembered the old Chinese proverb, "Be careful lest you get what you want."

Still not knowing what I wanted, I tried to look at the decision from a practical, financial point of view. The fertility drug protocol would cost several hundred dollars. The LTT, with my eggs or someone else's, would be $2000 to $4000 depending on the drugs used and the logistics. A private adoption would probably run between $5000 and $10,000, so if the operation worked the first time, it would certainly be the most cost-effective route. But if it didn't, we'd have nothing to show for it and that much less money available for adoption.

Money wasn't the real issue, however. I had to admit to myself that if I really wanted to make a baby and felt it was possible, I would come up with the resources somehow. The truth was that I found myself dreading the ordeal of more fertility treatment rather than being excited about the possible outcome. For whatever reason, I no longer felt a burning drive to bear a child. Had I given up? Little waves of guilt washed over me. Why wasn't I willing to go for it? Maybe I had just lost heart and hope temporarily; perhaps the will to press on was just dormant and in a week or two my faith and my enthusiasm would return. Talking about it with Bill one night, I decided to give myself until the end of the month to make up my mind.

During the month, we reminded each other periodically that a decision was due soon but had few conversations about it. The question of my commitment to bearing a child simmered inside me. Sometimes at night before sleeping, I would ask for a dream that would tell me what to do, but no clear message made it out of dreamland. I had almost forgotten my deadline on the afternoon of the thirty-first when I was talking with a single friend about the tyranny of the biological clock and about adoption. Alexander was playing across the room and I looked over at him pushing his plastic choo-choo train on yellow plastic tracks. It occurred to me suddenly, like a realization I had never had before (although I knew I had), that this little boy was everything I wanted in a biological child. He was blonde, blue-eyed, and beautiful. He looked like a little MaryBill and acted like us, too—happy and energetic, uncommonly friendly and open, quick to laugh and love. There was nothing missing in my experience of being a mother. My son was everything I wanted and more.

I had often said I felt the hand of God in our adoption of Alexander, indeed, in all the adoptions I had come to know. I felt ready to trust that God would again bring us the right child. Perhaps it would not be the girl we hoped for. Perhaps he or she would have dark hair, dark eyes, or dark skin. Perhaps our child would find us from another part of the world. We might be fortunate, as before, and find a baby easily, or we might have to work hard to adopt again and endure some trials. Whatever lay before us in finding our child, I felt ready to go at it with energy and enthusiasm.

In deciding not to pursue further fertility treatment I felt both relief and sadness. There was not the same wrenching grief as before, as my acceptance had grown gradually and had brought me resolution. Most fortunately, Bill shared in that resolution and in our dreams for the future of our family. We had endured a major life crisis and been strengthened— even blessed—by it. I knew that our infertility would always be with me, but not as an identity or an old wound. Instead, I would see it as a painful disability that we had overcome— not with medical technology but with the power of love.

Chapter Ten

❦

In Closing

*W*aiting for baby is a distinct time of life and a difficult one. At some point the waiting must end, and resolution, either happy or regretful, is achieved. Life goes on. The pain suffered fades as a child, children, or other interests fill the void. The suffering of those who experience infertility is not without its own consolations, however. Like any life crisis, it tests and strengthens, teaching us about parts of ourselves and our partners we might otherwise have no opportunity to know. In the process of coping with the pain of wanting what we can't have, we gain a degree of maturity. It is truly humbling to have to admit that you cannot control the forces of nature, not with all the technology of modern medicine at your disposal.

But while a little humility is a good thing, shame is not. There is no shame in the inability to conceive, any more than in other dysfunctions of the body. Nor does being unable to have a baby mean you are a failure or that you don't deserve happiness. People do not get pregnant because they are good or successful or deserving. Likewise, there is nothing wrong with people who do not get pregnant; we are just unlucky.

Until we resolve our situation, we unlucky ones are likely to be obsessed. The consuming passion to have a child tends to become the focus of our lives and gets in the way of enjoying life and being fully involved in all its aspects. Obsession is not a pretty picture, but it goes with the territory. And it's okay —for a while. How long a while depends on your emotional and financial stamina, and you will come to know your own limits. Keeping perspective in the throes of obsession seems impossible, but it can be done. You can step out of your infertile box every now and then and look about you. You are still alive, you are healthy, you have a life partner, and you have the resources to somehow, some way have a family, if that is what you desire, or to create a happy and fulfilling childfree future. This limbo will not last forever.

If you are able to keep the faith that you will have a family, you can enjoy life now rather than wait for a child to make you happy. I often think back to how unhappy I was during much of the time I was single. I was obsessed with finding a man to marry and worrying that it would never happen. Then when I found the right man, I started worrying right away about never having a baby. What a waste! I wish now I had been more relaxed about both developments in my life, that I had had faith, had trusted in the future, and had enjoyed fully what was on my plate at the moment. What is before you right now and what is your greatest asset is your relationship as a couple. Enjoy each other and this time alone together without the demands of family. Explore what it might mean for you to remain a family of two, and let that exploration contribute to resolving your infertility.

On the way to your resolution, you may discover, as Bill and I did, some valuable lessons for living. We found new opportunities to deepen our closeness by sharing our deepest fears and feelings. We learned how to listen to each other and how to console each other—when to offer solace and when to let the other be. We got better at expressing our feelings, both positive and negative, and learned to appreciate and accept our differences of opinion. Dealing with infertility also strengthened our sense of empathy and compassion—for each other and for other people. Many of us don't have the opportunity to feel truly needy, to know what it's like to have our dreams denied us. Compassion is passionate caring that expands our humility and our humanity.

Another by-product of our bout with infertility was greater clarity about the purpose and meaning of our lives, about what is truly important to us. We were profoundly grateful for the strength of our love for each other and for the loving support of our friends and families. We became even more certain that what we were here to do was share ourselves and our love and that we wanted a focus of that love to be our children. We found that other concerns, whether about money or status or freedom, were secondary to our commitment to family.

Of course, the greatest consolation prize of all was Alexander. I have often felt and said that I am glad for our infertility because it brought us Alexander. I don't know how a biological child could be more perfect or more loved, not because he is so "like us," but because he is so completely himself. Not a day passes that I don't feel incredibly blessed by his presence. I still marvel at the miraculous gift Eileen gave us and feel an everlasting gratitude. I have already recounted how deciding to adopt helped free me from some of the emotional chains of my own childhood and in the process, I believe, prepared me to be a more conscious and empowering mother. Letting go of the pictures of what I felt I must have —first in a man and then a baby—opened me up to receiving what life has to offer and finding it better than I could have imagined. Knowing that I can love another not of my blood strengthens my belief that we are one human family, possibly possessing the capacity to love ourselves out of the mess we've made.

The institution of adoption, with all its turmoil and change, is a blessed benefit of our society. While I don't think simplistically that adoption can replace abortion as a method of dealing with unwanted pregnancies, I certainly feel differently from how I once did about the choices we as a society provide for pregnant young women. Why should a young woman go through the ordeals of pregnancy and childbirth, perhaps losing her job as well as the respect of her family and friends, when she can easily get a ten-minute abortion? It isn't that she shouldn't have the choice to abort, but that some weight must be given to the alternatives. To the courageous women who do choose to carry a child, I feel society owes not only financial support, but moral support as well. I hope that carrying a baby and making a plan for its adoption will increasingly become a viable alternative to abortion. I hope that young women who feel pressure to keep babies they cannot support will see in adoption an honorable and magnanimous way to provide for their children.

It is also my hope that the climate for adoption in our society will continue to become more receptive and realistic. Just as birth mothers are still considered uncaring and callous for giving up their babies, adoptive parents and adopted children still face archaic attitudes that demean the adoption relationship. There is still the sentiment that an adopting couple has "settled for second best" and that the family is in for continuing problems. Birth parents are referred to as "the real parents," and adopted kids are made to feel different—a fate worse than death for a child. I look forward to a time when adoption will be seen for what it truly is—a life-enhancing opportunity for everyone in the triangle.

It now looks as if the pressures of the infertility "epidemic" will force changes in our adoption attitudes and policies. The rise in infertility may also begin to affect our priorities as women and as couples. When my friends in their early to mid-thirties tell me they plan to wait a few years to get pregnant, I find it difficult to say, as I once would have, "Sure, you've got plenty of time." I know how important it is for women to focus on their careers, particularly in these times when one income does not a mortgage make. But "baby-craving" (to borrow *Life* magazine's term) seems to be just as prevalent among women who dress for success. The bad news is that maybe we can't have it all, at least not in the time frame we'd like, that the forces of our biology are stronger than those of our will, that we can't fool Mother Nature. The best cure for infertility may be prevention, that is, not ignoring our peak fertility period in favor of freedom, independence, and career. As more women try to balance the demands of being a wage earner with those of starting a family, our society will need to respond with a great deal more support, from day care to paid parental leave to flexible working situations.

These various thoughts about the future of infertility and adoption may seem far from your concerns now. You may be more interested in what new treatment opportunities are developing—what is going to get you pregnant. By all means, keep up your energy to try what is feasible for you. Scientific knowledge increases exponentially, and the young science of infertility holds much promise for more effective, less invasive, and less expensive treatment. Go after that treatment aggressively and knowledgably, taking responsibility, along with your doctor, for seeing that it is appropriate for you. Remember that your doctor does not possess a magic wand, but something he or she does or you do or the Almighty does may bring you a baby.

If God, man, or medicine doesn't produce a child for

you, perhaps another woman will. Adoption isn't second best, it is only another path to creating a family. I feel about it as another adoptive couple once stated: "God doesn't always give you what you want. Sometimes God gives you something better."

❦

Resources and Books on Infertility and Adoption

INFERTILITY

Organizations

RESOLVE, INC.
National Office
5 Water St.
Arlington, MA 02174
(617) 643-2424

National self-help organization for infertile couples. Provides information, education, referrals, and a newsletter. Local RESOLVE chapters throughout the U.S. offer support groups and referrals.

AMERICAN FERTILITY SOCIETY
2140 11th Avenue South, Suite 200
Birmingham, AL 35205-2800
(205) 933-8494

National organization for health professionals specializing in fertility. Provides referrals and publishes a monthly journal.

AMERICAN COLLEGE OF OBSTETRICS AND GYNECOLOGY
600 Maryland Avenue S.W., Suite 300
Washington, D.C. 20024
Professional organization providing lists of infertility specialists.

General Infertility Books

Andrew, Lori B., J.D. *New Conceptions: A Consumer's Guide to the Newest Infertility Treatments.* New York: St. Martin's Press, 1984.

Bellina, Joseph H., M.D., Ph.D., and Wilson, Josleen. *You CAN Have a Baby.* New York: Crown, 1985.

Harkness, Carla. *The Infertility Book: A Comprehensive Medical and Emotional Guide.* San Francisco: Volcano Press, 1987.

Liebmann-Smith, Joan. *In Pursuit of Pregnancy: How Couples Discover, Cope With, and Resolve Their Fertility Problems.* New York: Newmarket Press, 1987.

Mazor, Miriam D., M.D., and Simons, Harriet F., eds. *Infertility: Medical, Emotional and Social Considerations.* New York: Human Sciences Press, 1984.

Menning, Barbara Eck. *Infertility: A Guide for the Childless Couple.* New York: Prentice-Hall, 1988 (second edition).

Salzer, Linda. *Infertility: How Couples Can Cope.* Boston: G.K. Hall, 1986.

Silber, Sherman, M.D. *How to Get Pregnant.* New York: Warner Books, 1981.

Stangel, John J., M.D. *Fertility and Conception: An Essential Guide for Childless Couples.* New York: North American Publishing, 1980.

Stephenson, Linda Rutledge. *Give Us A Child: Coping with the Personal Crisis of Infertility.* San Francisco: Harper & Row, Publishers, 1987.

Books on Other Issues

Berg, Susan, and Lasker, Judith. *When Pregnancy Fails: Coping with Miscarriage, Stillbirth, and Infant Death.* Boston: Beacon Press, 1981.

Friedman, Rochelle, M.D., and Gradstein, Bonnie. *Surviving Pregnancy Loss.* Boston: Little, Brown and Co., 1982.

Noble, Elizabeth. *Having Your Baby by Donor Insemination: The Complete Resource Guide.* Boston: Houghton Mifflin Co., 1987.

Older, Julia A. *A Woman's Guide to Endometriosis.* New York: Charles Scribner's Sons, 1984.

Tilton, Nan and Tom, and Moore, Gaylen. *Making Miracles: In Vitro Fertilization.* Garden City, N.Y.: Doubleday, 1985.

Overvald, Amy Zuckerman. *Surrogate Parenting.* New York: Pharos Books, 1988.

Faux, Marian. *Childless by Choice: Choosing Childlessness in the Eighties.* New York: Doubleday, 1984.

Bombardieri, Merle, *The Baby Decision: How to Make the Most Important Choice of Your Life.* New York: Rawson, Wade Publishers Inc., 1981. (Order from author at 26 Trapelo Rd., Belmont, MA 02178, $12.45 paper, $18.45 hardcover, including shipping and handling.)

ADOPTION

Organizations

NATIONAL COMMITTEE FOR ADOPTION
1346 Connecticut Ave. N.W., Suite 326
Washington, D.C. 20036
(202) 463-7559

Provides information and referrals.

OURS, INC.
3307 Highway 100 North, Suite 203
Minneapolis, MN 55442
(612) 535-4829

Provides information, referrals, and a newsletter about international adoption.

NATIONAL FEDERATION OF INDEPENDENT AND OPEN ADOPTION CENTERS
3333 Vincent Road, Suite 222
Pleasant Hill, CA 94523-4353
(415) 944-4744

Provides information and referrals and publishes *The New Adoption Journal* on independent and open adoption.

Books on Adoption

Arms, Suzanne. *To Love and Let Go*. New York: Alfred A. Knopf, 1983.

Canape, Charlene. *Adoption: Parenthood Without Pregnancy*. New York: Henry Holt and Co., 1986.

Gilman, Lois. *The Adoption Resource Book*. New York: Harper & Row, Publishers, 1984.

Lindsay, Jeanne Warren. *Open Adoption: A Caring Option*. Buena Park, Cal.: Morning Glory Press, 1987.

Martin, Cynthia D., Ph.D. *Beating the Adoption Game*. San Diego: Harcourt Brace Jovanovich, Publishers, 1988 (revised).

Melina, Lois Ruskai. *Raising Adopted Children*. New York: Harper & Row, Publishers, 1986.

Plumez, Jacqueline H. *Successful Adoption: A Guide to Finding a Child and Raising a Family*. New York: Crown Publishers, 1982.

Rillera, Mary Jo, and Kaplan, Sharon. *Cooperative Adoption: A Handbook*. Westminster, Cal.: Triadoption Publications, 1984.

Silber, Kathleen, and Speedlin, Phylis. *Dear Birthmother*. San Antonio: Corona Publishing Co., 1983.

Sorosky, Arthur D., M.D., Baran, Annette, and Pannor, Reuben. *The Adoption Triangle*. Garden City, N.Y.: Anchor Books, 1984 (revised).

Viguers, Susan T. *With Child: One Couple's Journey to Their Adopted Children*. San Diego: Harcourt Brace Jovanovich, Publishers, 1986.